Acclaim for
*What Your Doctor May Not Tell You About
Heart Disease*

"If you think taking a statin or blood pressure pill will protect you against heart disease, think again. Dr. Mark Houston's groundbreaking book explains the *real* causes of heart disease and provides a practical set of tools to uncover your hidden heart disease risks, and a road map to a healthy heart. Sadly, we are missing the boat on heart disease, but Dr. Houston takes us on a steamship to the future of prevention, treatment, and reversal of heart disease. If you have a heart, read this book."

—Mark Hyman, MD, *New York Times* bestselling
author of *The UltraMind Solution* and *UltraMetabolism*

"If you're interested in knowing the real truth about heart disease, you must read this book! Dr. Houston cuts through all the myths and misconceptions and tells you exactly what to do to keep your heart healthy. A superb addition to any library!"

—Jonny Bowden, PhD, CNS, bestselling author of
The 150 Healthiest Foods on Earth and
The Most Effective Ways to Live Longer

"Do you wish you had more of your doctor's time to discuss your health? Then this book is your prescription. Do tell your doctor you are using food and nutrients against heart disease. Your doctor is likely to augment your efforts and reduce your prescription medications, because cardiologist Dr. Mark Houston's protocols work."

—Ingrid Kohlstadt, MD, MPH, FACN, FACPM,
editor of *Food and Nutrients in Disease Management*

"Dr. Mark Houston has written a very fine book. His discussion of cholesterol is absolutely outstanding. He dispels the myth and dissects the science utilizing targeted nutraceuticals that absolutely work. A brilliant portrayal! This book is a must-read for anyone taking a statin drug or especially for those who are overly concerned about their cholesterol and their heart."

—Stephen T. Sinatra, MD, FACC, FACN,
author of *The Sinatra Solution*

"Ignorance is not bliss when it comes to our health...Learning the truth behind coronary illness as found in Dr. Mark Houston's latest 'user-friendly' book may very well save your life! Feast on facts about how you can make informed choices that not only affect you, but those you love...A heartfelt thanks, Dr. Mark!"

—Jennifer O'Neill, model, actress, author, and speaker

"Want to reduce the cost of health care by 50 percent four years from now? Make this groundbreaking book mandatory reading for all medical students in the summer *prior* to entering medical school. They will realize that much of what is assumed as being risk factors for cardiovascular disease is misleading... The biggest advantage is [that] the reader is given attack plans that will customize the healing processes that will optimize the cardiovascular system. Another plus is the section on exercise...Make sure to give your physician his/her own copy, because after all, doctors listen to doctors."

—Charles Poliquin, strength coach of Olympic medalists in seventeen different sports

"The world needs more pioneers like Dr. Houston! The hard truths in this book will save millions of lives—and blow the tired old myths on cholesterol and heart disease right out of the water. This is a must-read for every human being on the planet who wants to steer clear of heart disease."

—Esther Blum, MS, RD, CDN, CNS, author of
Eat, Drink, and Be Gorgeous, Secrets of Gorgeous and
The Eat, Drink, and Be Gorgeous Project

"Preventing heart disease is much more than 'managing' your cholesterol, eating a low-fat diet, or taking a statin medication...Dr. Houston presents an interesting and provocative case for expanding our thinking about heart health. An important read for anyone looking to protect their cardiovascular system and improve their well-being."

"This book is filled with the real risk factors for heart disease and what you can do to lower your own risk for a heart attack. I recommend you tell everyone about this book. It could save your life."

"In a clear and concise style, Houston dispels the myths surrounding heart disease and opens our eyes to the true role of the traditional cardiac risk factors...Houston pushes cardiology into the twenty-first century. His expanded and integrative approach is a must-read for practitioners as well as patients."

WHAT YOUR DOCTOR MAY *NOT* TELL YOU ABOUT®

HEART DISEASE

Also by Mark C. Houston, MD, MS

What Your Doctor May Not *Tell You About Hypertension*

Handbook of Hypertension

Hypertension Handbook for Students and Clinicians

Handbook of Hypertension

WHAT YOUR DOCTOR MAY NOT TELL YOU ABOUT®

HEART DISEASE

The Revolutionary Book That Reveals
the Truth Behind Coronary Illnesses—
And How You Can Fight Them

MARK C. HOUSTON, MD, MS

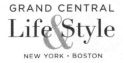

GRAND CENTRAL
Life & Style
NEW YORK • BOSTON

Copyright © 2012 by Mark Houston, MD

Grand Central Life & Style
Hachette Book Group
237 Park Avenue
New York, NY 10017

www.GrandCentralLifeandStyle.com

Printed in the United States of America

First Edition: February 2012
10 9 8 7 6 5 4

Grand Central Life & Style is an imprint of Grand Central Publishing.
The Grand Central Life & Style name and logo are trademarks of Hachette Book Group, Inc.

The Hachette Speakers Bureau provides a wide range of authors for speaking events. To find out more, go to www.hachettespeakersbureau.com or call (866) 376-6591.

The publisher is not responsible for websites (or their content) that are not owned by the publisher.

Library of Congress Cataloging-in-Publication Data

Houston, Mark C.
What your doctor may not tell you about heart disease / by Mark C. Houston. — 1st ed.
p. cm.
ISBN 978-1-60941-254-8
1. Heart—Diseases—Popular works.   2. Heart—Diseases—Treatment—Popular works.
I. Title.
RC672.H68 2012
616.1'2—dc23

2011023237

This book is dedicated to my loving family and my God. To my wife, Laurie; my four children, Helen, Bo, John, and Kelly; my mother, Mary Ruth Houston; and my father, R. R. Houston. I also want to thank all of my wonderful friends, mentors, and patients over the years. I have been blessed by all of these people, and without their support and love, I would not have achieved all that I have in this life.

Contents

Acknowledgments

I could not have written this book without the assistance of Esther Blum, MS, RD, CDN, CNS, who provided nutrition information, and Charles Poliquin, strength coach; and Jade Teta, ND, CSCS, and Mick Weber, MS, CCN, who taught me much about exercise.

WHAT YOUR DOCTOR MAY *NOT* TELL YOU ABOUT®

HEART DISEASE

Introduction

I<small>T'S A SAD</small> story that's repeated thousands of times every year. A person, let's say an overweight fifty-seven-year-old man named Bruce, gets the bad news from his doctor following a routine physical examination: "Your total cholesterol is 235, which is a little high, and your LDL cholesterol, that's the 'bad' cholesterol, is also a bit high at 160." The "good" news then follows: "I'm going to prescribe a medicine that will lower those numbers and keep your heart safe."

Bruce gladly takes the medicine, confident that doing so will add years to his life by preventing him from developing heart disease or having a heart attack. And indeed, both his total cholesterol and LDL cholesterol levels quickly drop into the "safe" range. But five years later, Bruce suffers a major heart attack, becoming another victim of coronary heart disease, long the number-one killer in this country. And he also becomes another victim of the heart attack myth.

Most heart attacks are caused by coronary heart disease (also known as coronary artery disease). Plaque, a sticky substance made up of fatty material, oxidized cholesterol and fats, inflammatory cells, immune cells, and other substances, builds up inside the arteries and eventually ruptures (literally explodes). This causes the formation of a blood clot inside the arteries that can slow or even stop the flow of blood to a portion of the heart. Depending on the severity of the blockage, a dizzying array of signs and symptoms may arise, including abnormal heartbeat, fluid in the lungs, shortness of breath, chest pain on exertion, chronic fatigue, dizziness, swollen feet and ankles, congestive heart failure, and, everyone's biggest nightmare, a heart attack or even sudden death.

For decades, you have been told that five risk factors are linked to almost all cases of coronary heart disease: elevated cholesterol, high blood pressure, diabetes mellitus, obesity, and smoking. You've also been told (directly or indirectly) that if these five are kept under control, you're practically guaranteed *not* to have a heart attack. And, quite frankly, *that's a lie.* The truth of the matter is this:

- Abnormal cholesterol levels are *not* primary causes or indicators of coronary heart disease.
- Consuming a high-cholesterol diet or eating eggs does *not* significantly raise blood cholesterol levels for most people.
- All LDL "bad" cholesterol is *not* harmful and does not necessarily cause coronary heart disease.
- All HDL "good" cholesterol is *not* protective—some types may actually be harmful and *promote* coronary heart disease.
- The blood pressure reading taken in your physician's office may *not* be an accurate measure of your true blood pressure.
- A fasting morning blood sugar reading of 99 mg/dL, deemed normal by most labs, is *not* safe or normal. Instead, it indicates an increased risk of coronary heart disease and heart attack.
- A normal body weight (as indicated by the scale) does *not* ensure heart health, as it doesn't reflect the amount of the risky visceral, or "belly," fat that promotes heart disease.

I have seen many patients who have what the lab considers "normal" cholesterol, blood pressure, and blood sugar levels lying flat on their backs in the coronary intensive care unit. For example:

Matt was forty-five years old and had a total cholesterol reading of 190 mg/dL, a blood sugar reading of 95 mg/dL, and a blood pressure reading of 122/78 mm Hg, all of which were "normal" and supposedly good numbers. Matt was not overweight and did not smoke, yet he had just been rushed to the hospital with a mild heart attack.

Jane, age fifty-two, was at her ideal body weight, had never smoked cigarettes, and had a total cholesterol level of 174 mg/dL and an LDL of 98 mg/dL (again, "good" numbers). Her blood pressure was in the safe range, at 110/76 mm Hg, and her blood sugar was considered normal at 98 mg/dL. Yet she suffered a severe heart attack that left her heart so weak, almost any physical effort was too taxing.

Sixty-year-old Tom had a total cholesterol of 158 mg/dL, an LDL cholesterol of 88 mg/dL, and an HDL cholesterol of 42 mg/dL. His blood pressure reading was 124/82 mm Hg, and his blood sugar was 92 mg/dL. Tom was not overweight and did not use any tobacco products. He seemed perfectly healthy, yet one day, seemingly out of the blue, his heart was struck with a fatal arrhythmia.

"How could I have had a heart attack?" patients with test results like these have asked me. "My cholesterol is good, my blood pressure is good, and my blood sugar is good! What went wrong? What's the real story about these numbers and the risk factors?"

The startling truth is that these factors are *not* the heart disease villains you've been led to believe they are. Take cholesterol, for example. The present preoccupation with keeping the numbers for total cholesterol—LDL, HDL, and blood fats (triglycerides)—within a certain range ignores new discoveries about the true role of cholesterol in heart disease.

- You may have total cholesterol and LDL cholesterol levels high enough to make your physician panic, yet still have fairly healthy arteries.
- You may have normal total cholesterol or LDL cholesterol levels that would not worry your doctor at all, yet have very unhealthy arteries.
- You may have a very high level of HDL "good" cholesterol, yet still have an increased risk of developing coronary heart disease.

Why? Because coronary heart disease doesn't come from cholesterol; it is the result of inflammation, oxidative stress (free radical damage), and autoimmune damage to your coronary arteries and other arteries throughout your body. Similarly, it's not the elevated blood glucose that "kills" your arteries or even the pounding of the blood against the blood vessel walls seen in high blood pressure; it's the inflammation, oxidative stress, and faulty immune response that may result. These are the elements you should be attempting to control. And taking medications to lower your cholesterol, blood sugar, or blood pressure will not necessarily accomplish these aims. In fact, they may open the door to disaster by giving you and your physician a false sense of security. Indeed, many recent papers published in medical journals have noted that addressing only the five major risk factors for coronary heart disease will never prevent or control nearly as much disease as we'd like. In other words, if doctors continue to focus almost exclusively on these five factors, we'll never do any better than we do now at treating coronary heart disease and heart attack!

In this book, I will explain the *true* risk factors for coronary heart disease, explain how you can discover which of these factors is threatening your heart health, and tell you how to lower or eliminate the risk(s) through proper nutrition, nutritional supplements, exercise, and other methods. You may not get this information from your doctor—he or she either doesn't know about it or doesn't have the time to explain it to you. And what your doctor may not tell you (or may not even know) about heart disease can be deadly. The pages that follow contain vital information that just might save your life.

Chapter One

The *Real* Reason People Have Heart Attacks

THIS IS A BOOK about coronary heart disease, which comes about when the arteries that carry fresh blood to the heart are blocked and the flow of fresh blood to a portion of the heart drops dramatically or ceases entirely. Depending on the extent of the blockage, the result can be anything from the chest pain of angina to a sudden and fatal heart attack. Although a number of other problems can afflict the heart, including faulty valves, coronary heart disease is what most people think about when someone says "heart disease."

Most doctors talk about coronary heart disease prevention as if it were a matter of dodging five "bullets," namely:

- elevated cholesterol (specifically LDL "bad" cholesterol)
- high blood pressure
- diabetes mellitus
- obesity
- smoking

This focus on the "Big Five" risk factors is all pervasive; you've probably even seen those "How Long Will You Live?" equations that supposedly calculate the power these risk factors have to induce coronary heart disease. The equations contain instructions like "Subtract 6 points if your cholesterol is over 300" and "Add 2 points if you don't smoke." These may be fun to play with, but they are misleading because they don't address the real causes of heart disease.

I prefer to think of the evolution of heart disease as a trip through a giant maze. When you first enter the Heart Disease Maze, you see hundreds of little pathways that wander all over the place, leading nowhere in particular. The walls lining these pathways are low, and there's plenty of light, so you experience no feeling of urgency or danger; instead, you feel as if you can safely wander from path to path forever. These paths represent the hundreds of biochemical and other variations in your body that are often small and, by themselves, don't matter. But if one variation is joined by others, you may find yourself on the fast track to heart disease. Examples of these variations include your blood levels of C-reactive protein, the size and number of your LDL cholesterol particles, the type and blood level of the fat known as triglyceride, your blood level of homocysteine, the type and size of HDL "good" cholesterol, your blood level of tumor necrosis factor (a marker of inflammation), and your blood level of interleukin-6 (a protein molecule that regulates the immune system). A few variations, such as uric acid levels, are routinely measured in standard blood tests; many others can be determined through specialized blood work or other tests. These variations also include certain diseases, such as chronic obstructive pulmonary disease, and infections, such as *H. pylori*, that by themselves don't lead to heart disease.

But back to the maze: If you just strolled down a few of these paths for a while, then hopped over the short walls and walked out of the Heart Disease Maze, all would be well. However, if you kept walking and followed too many paths, or followed one or more for too long, you would suddenly realize that you were moving along a different kind of path—one with higher walls, less light, and a kind of spooky feeling. You would have moved from the innocuous "Variations Pathways" to one of the considerably more dangerous "Fast Track to Heart Disease Pathways." You wouldn't have noticed any signs indicating you were leaving the little Variations Pathways and entering the ominous Fast Track to Heart Disease Pathways, but there you'd be.

For many people, the Fast Track Pathways of greatest concern are the following seven:

- Inflammation Pathway
- Oxidative Stress Pathway
- Vascular Autoimmune Pathway
- Dyslipidemia Pathway
- Blood Pressure Pathway
- Blood Sugar Pathway
- Obesity and Increased Body Fat Pathway

Once you're on a Fast Track to Heart Disease Pathway, you'll find yourself moving faster and faster into darker, spookier territory. You'd like to stop but don't know how, because there are no road signs or helpful people telling you how to get off. There are some doors in the very high walls that would let you out of the maze, but they're difficult to spot unless you know what you're looking for. Odds are you'll keep moving ahead until you find yourself on the very dark and frightening "Faulty Arteries Pathway," hurtling forward into the darkness. Even then there are a few ladders propped up against the very high walls that you could use to climb out of there, but they're very hard to spot and grab hold of. That's why there is a very good chance you'll continue speeding forward in the darkness until you slam headlong into the brick wall called a heart attack.

This may be an oversimplified way of looking at the development of coronary heart disease and heart attacks, but it illustrates an important point: the disease process typically starts innocently with small problems having to do with inflammation, oxidative stress, or the way the immune system functions in the arteries (vascular autoimmunity)—a few minor variations in the levels of substances that most doctors don't measure or even connect with heart disease. I call them variations because they're often not out-and-out problems or diseases; they're just a bit too much or too little of a measurable substance or the presence of a certain state. But when they're combined with others, they can become troublesome. Even then they may not hurt you, thanks to your unique biochemistry and other factors. But if you have the wrong combination of genetics and other factors, you'll need to slam on the brakes and get off that road as soon as possible, or your journey may come to an abrupt and unfortunate end, because now you have early-stage disease of the arteries, and they're not working the way they should.

As a hypertension and vascular specialist practicing preventive cardiology, I've been frustrated by the fact that most people have no idea they're in the Heart Disease Maze until they're already on the Faulty Arteries Pathway or have splattered into the brick wall at the end of the journey. If only they knew how easy it is to step out of the maze at the beginning of the journey or how to get off the Fast Track to Heart Disease and Faulty Arteries Pathways or, better yet, how to avoid them altogether. But they don't know because they're not told these things by their physicians.

That's going to change, starting now. In this book, I'll introduce you to hundreds of biochemical and other changes (technically called risk mediators and risk factors) that make up the Variations Pathways, as well as several of the Fast Tracks to Heart Disease—inflammation, oxidative stress, vascular autoimmune dysfunction, dyslipidemia, disturbances to blood pressure and flow, and problems with blood sugar—that arise when variations interact with one's unique body chemistry and lifestyle. But first, let's take a look at the terrifying Faulty Arteries Pathway (technically called endothelial dysfunction) that inevitably results from these Fast Tracks—a pathway traveled by virtually everyone who has a heart attack.

THE ENDOTHELIUM: WHERE TROUBLE IN THE ARTERIES BEGINS

The cardiovascular system consists of a heart that pumps blood and the blood vessels that carry the blood to all parts of the body, then return it to the heart. The blood vessels that carry blood away from the heart are called arteries; those that carry it toward the heart are called veins. It's the arteries that we're concerned with when we speak about cardiovascular disease. Most people think of the arteries as something akin to the water pipes in a house—all they do is carry water from the street, through the house, and back out. Like water pipes, they believe, arteries are inert little tubes that have no influence on the fluid they carry or the pump that keeps that fluid moving. Nothing could be further from the truth.

Unlike the water pipes in your house, arteries are complex, multilayered, living tubes that do much more than transport fluid. The arteries and their smaller versions, the arterioles, carry freshly oxygenated blood from the heart to all parts of the body. But they also perform many tasks to ensure that the blood keeps flowing at the right speed and physical consistency, and in the correct manner. If they fail to perform correctly, the consequences can be severe.

As you can see in Figure 1, the artery is a complex structure

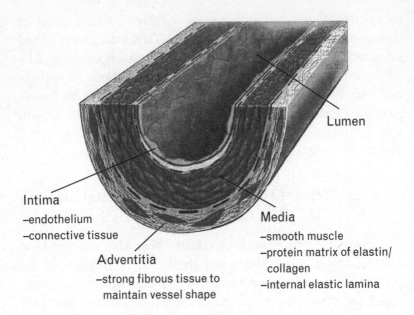

Lumen

Intima
–endothelium
–connective tissue

Media
–smooth muscle
–protein matrix of elastin/
 collagen
–internal elastic lamina

Adventitia
–strong fibrous tissue to
 maintain vessel shape

Figure 1: The Arterial Wall

made up of several layers of tissues, each with its own duties and characteristics.

The central part of the artery, the open area through which blood flows, is called the lumen. This is the corridor through which the blood travels, with its red blood cells, white blood cells, platelets, proteins, nutrients, oxygen, and numerous other substances.

The layer that the blood actually comes into contact with is called the intima. It's made up of the endothelium, which serves as the smooth inner lining of the vessel, plus connective tissue. The endothelium is the tissue in which coronary heart disease originates.

Moving deeper into the arterial wall, we come to the media, a thicker layer made up of smooth muscle that contracts and relaxes at the appropriate times, which helps control the flow of blood and the pressure. The outer layer, called the adventitia, is made up of connective tissues that help the artery maintain its shape and prevent it from bulging outward.

The endothelium, the point of contact between blood and artery, is very thin—just one cell deep. It has a variety of duties, including:

- *acting as a barrier* by allowing only specific substances to pass from the blood into the artery
- *fighting off disease and regulating the way the immune system behaves in the artery* by producing interleukins and other substances that play important roles in the battle against bacteria and other dangers
- *regulating blood pressure* and arterial tone by synthesizing substances such as angiotensin converting enzyme, angiotensin II, nitric oxide, and endothelin, which help regulate blood pressure
- *controlling inflammation and oxidative stress*
- *maintaining homeostasis* and controlling the growth of arteries by detecting and responding to changes in the oxygen content of blood, as well as other indicators of the blood's status and composition
- *fine-tuning the blood* and helping to keep it thin and fluid enough to flow easily through the blood vessels
- *controlling blood clotting*

As you can see, the endothelium is much more than an inert pipe. If it is damaged, you will find yourself on the road to heart disease and may suffer from numerous other ailments as well. Even if you're thin, a nonsmoker, and have great cholesterol levels and low blood pressure, if your endothelium is damaged, you're in trouble.

Because the endothelium produces substances that alter the actions of the arteries and makes "executive decisions" about which substances are allowed to pass through it, the endothelium qualifies as an organ and is, in fact, the largest organ in the body. If you took it out of the arteries, flattened it, and laid it out, it would cover six and a half tennis courts!

Even though the endothelium is the "brain" of the arteries, it is not encased in a protective sheath or buried safely within the artery wall. Instead, it is in direct contact with the bacteria, hormones, and other substances in the blood that can either harm it or alter its behavior. And it is right up against the pounding of the blood that continuously rushes through the arteries, like a beach subjected to the forces of heavy waves, twenty-four hours a day. While it may not matter whether a beach is reshaped by the ceaseless action of the water, the endothelium cannot allow itself to be altered by the tremendous force of the blood flowing past. It must maintain its structural and functional integrity. Unfortunately, it can't always do that.

THE GENERAL EFFECTS OF A DAMAGED ENDOTHELIUM

When the endothelium is damaged, its ability to serve as an intelligent barrier between the blood and the arteries is compromised. We call this condition *endothelial dysfunction*. When this occurs, several things can happen. The wrong substances— LDL cholesterol, white blood cells called monocytes, and other immune system cells and proteins—may pass from the blood into the arterial wall. The endothelium may over- or underproduce key mediators, substances, or hormones. Its ability to keep blood viscosity at the right level may falter, possibly allowing the blood to become thick, sluggish, and more likely to clot inappropriately. And since the endothelium is responsible for releasing substances that relax the arterial muscles and help regulate blood flow, the arteries may become constricted. This can cause blood pressure to rise and, depending on where the constriction is, blood flow to the heart to decrease.

Endothelial dysfunction leads to many problems with the arteries themselves, including

- thickening of the endothelium (which should only be one cell thick) and the arterial wall
- increased arterial inflammation
- increased oxidative stress (free radical damage)
- autoimmune dysfunction of the artery (the immune system mistakenly attacks the arteries)
- increased deposits of protein, fats, and inflammatory cells into the artery walls

As damage to the endothelium accumulates and intensifies, the entire artery may become stiff, blocked, or otherwise ineffectual. Unfortunately, the problems triggered by endothelial dysfunction can make the condition worse, setting in motion a vicious circle and an intensification of the disease. For example, problems with the endothelium can make it impossible for the arteries to relax at the appropriate times, elevating the blood pressure. As blood pressure rises, the extra force exerted by the blood can further damage the endothelium and increase the endothelial dysfunction—which makes blood pressure rise even higher.

There are more than four hundred biochemical and biomechanical mediators of endothelial dysfunction—that is, things that can harm the endothelium. That's an almost infinite number of insults the endothelium and artery may suffer, but there are only a finite number of responses, or things the endothelium and artery can do to protect themselves when they're harmed. These responses are to trigger inflammation, oxidative stress, and autoimmune dysfunction of the arteries. These are standard "weapons" the body uses when attacked, but, unfortunately, they can make the problem worse, leading to endothelial dysfunction, abnormal arterial stiffness, and a lack of compliance, or the ability of the arteries to bend and relax in response to changing conditions.

ENDOTHELIAL DYSFUNCTION AND HEART DISEASE

For years we believed that heart disease began with atherosclerosis ("clogged arteries"), a process initiated when excess cholesterol and fat in the bloodstream stuck to the inner lining of an artery. More and more stuck and eventually blocked the flow of blood in an artery supplying the heart, triggering a heart attack. That idea is now obsolete. Today we understand that heart disease begins with an injury to the endothelium. Think of this injury as a microscopic scratch, like a paper cut on your finger that you can't even see. Many things may have caused the scratch, including substances in cigarette smoke, elevated levels of glucose (sugar) or homocysteine in the bloodstream, chronic infections. toxins or heavy metals, oxidized LDL cholesterol, elevated blood pressure, or sheer stress on the arterial wall.

While you or I would probably ignore an insignificant scratch, the body is much more thorough. It triggers the inflammation process, rushing white blood cells, platelets, and other immune cells to the injured area to patch things up. But these immune cells don't simply slap a kind of "molecular bandage" on the scratch and leave. Instead, some of these cells bind to the site, while others burrow through the endothelium and into the artery wall. These immune system cells, along with small, dense LDL cholesterol (which becomes oxidized and

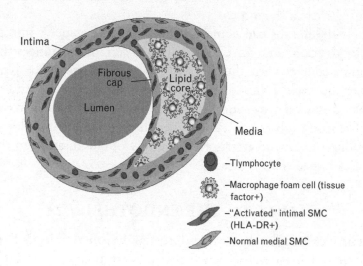

Intima

Fibrous
cap

Lipid
core

Lumen

Media

-Tlymphocyte

-Macrophage foam cell (tissue
 factor+)

-"Activated" intimal SMC
 (HLA-DR+)

-Normal medial SMC

Figure 2: The Anatomy of Atherosclerotic Plaque

modified), smooth muscle cells, inflammatory cells, cytokines, chemokines, and clotting substances combine to form a toxic brew within the inner artery wall. It's like an improvised explosive device buried in one of the walls of your arteries.

The toxic brew is walled off from the bloodstream. But it is not harmless, for it sends out signals that increase inflammation, oxidative stress, and harmful autoimmune activity. With time, the toxic brew inside the artery wall grows larger and more dangerous and becomes covered by a fibrous cap—a sort of arterial scab. If the toxic brew is large enough, it may cause the intima to bulge inward, interfering with the flow of blood. But even if a bulge grows large enough to block 50, 60, or even 80 percent of the passageway, it may not cause a problem. Even obstructions of 98 percent may be relatively asymptomatic—

unless the fibrous cap ruptures or is ripped off, which is the thing we fear the most.

If the fibrous cap comes off, the toxic brew spews into the bloodstream. The toxic brew contains certain substances that, upon contact with the blood, cause an instantaneous blood clot. So even if a coronary artery is completely clear and the blood has been flowing through it freely, that sudden release of clotting substances can trigger the formation of a clot big enough to fill the artery, stop the flow of blood, and cause an instantaneous heart attack.

LOOK TO THE ENDOTHELIUM

There's no doubt about it: endothelial dysfunction leads to the arterial damage that's a key factor in heart disease, even if there is no elevated cholesterol, no signs of "hardening of the arteries," and no evidence of high blood pressure. That's why simply taking medicines that lower cholesterol or blood pressure, or counteract elevated blood sugar, is not the answer if your endothelium is malfunctioning.

Ron, a forty-two-year-old man, was rushed to the emergency room when he complained of chest pain. He told the doctors that he had been having "moderate" chest pain off and on for several months. Ron, who was severely overweight, also divulged that he smoked a pack of cigarettes every day and was under a lot of stress. He was given the standard tests, which revealed that he had elevated levels of total cholesterol, LDL "bad" cholesterol, blood pressure, and fasting blood sugar. However, his cardiac angiogram showed that his coronary arteries were all "wide open," with only minimal blockages. (That's not surprising, for toxic brews can be hidden in the arterial walls and not protrude much into the lumen.) Ron's doctors assured him that he was fine and just needed to stop smoking, lose weight, take medicines to control his cholesterol, and otherwise keep his Big Five risk factors under control.

Ron was an excellent patient and took his medicines exactly as prescribed. He also lost 20 pounds and cut back from one pack to half a pack of cigarettes a day. At his regular check-ups, his doctor was delighted. Then, three years later, Ron had his first heart attack.

He was sent to see me, and the tests I performed showed significant damage to the endothelium—which could have been detected earlier, had someone looked. If Ron had worked to reduce the factors that contributed to his endothelial dysfunction, he probably wouldn't have had that heart attack.

Let me be clear: I don't mean to imply that it's okay to have elevated cholesterol, blood pressure, or blood sugar, or to smoke or be obese. But our decades-long insistence that the Big Five are the be-all and end-all of heart disease is a tragic myth that has led millions to an early grave. Endothelial dysfunction is much more important than any of these factors.

HOW DO YOU KNOW IF YOU HAVE ENDOTHELIAL DYSFUNCTION?

Endothelial dysfunction can be detected easily by several tests performed in the doctor's office. They are accurate, giving a clear indication of the risk of coronary heart disease. They are also noninvasive, relatively inexpensive, and take less than fifteen minutes to complete. They include the following tests:

- *Computerized Arterial Pulse Waveform Analysis (CAPWA)*— This test measures the elasticity of large and small arteries (their ability to widen and narrow in reaction to the pulsing of the blood). A poor result means the arteries are stiffer than they should be, indicating early endothelial dysfunction. A CAPWA is quick and simple; small monitors attached to the body feed information to a computer over the course of ten minutes. The patient simply lies on a table during the test.

- *EndoPAT*—This test monitors the flow of blood, the relationship between blood flow in the arms and fingers, and the changes that occur as a blood pressure cuff on one arm is inflated and deflated. The results from the arm with the cuff are compared with those from the other arm to determine endothelial health.

- *Digital Thermal Monitoring (DTM)*—DTM measures the ability of the arteries to widen and narrow by monitoring temperature. (Blood is warm, so changes in blood flow in the tiny blood vessels in the fingertips slightly alter the fingertip temperature, making fingertip temperature a surrogate measurement for blood flow.) A blood pressure cuff is attached to the arm, inflated to interfere with blood flow to the fingers, then deflated to allow the flow to return to normal. Changes in fingertip temperature allow the doctors to gauge endothelial health.

- *Carotid Artery Duplex Scan*—This painless test uses ultrasound waves to generate a computerized "snapshot" of the blood flowing through the carotid arteries and identify any thickening, narrowing, or obstructions.

- *Ankle-Brachial Index (ABI)*—This test compares blood flow in the ankle to blood flow in the brachial artery of the arm before and after exercise (walking on a treadmill for five minutes). Normally, the blood pressure at your ankle should be equal to or a little higher than the pressure in your arm, producing an ankle-brachial index or ratio of about 0.9 to 1.3. Deviations from this average suggest trouble in the arteries.

- *Carotid Intimal Medial Thickness (IMT)*—This test uses ultrasound to measure the thickness of the intima and media of the carotid arteries, which run through the neck. As blood pressure increases and a toxic brew forms within a damaged artery, its walls become thicker. Thickening of the carotid arteries has been shown to be a strong indicator of cardiovascular disease and atherosclerosis. It also signals an increased risk of coronary heart disease, heart attack, and stroke.

Based on the results of these and perhaps other tests, your physician will be able to determine whether you are suffering from endothelial dysfunction and, if you are, to what degree. If you have signs of endothelial dysfunction, you need to take action now, because you're on the Faulty Arteries Pathway, which can easily cause a heart attack or stroke. If you don't show signs of endothelial dysfunction, you're not necessarily in the clear, as you might still be on one of the Fast Track to Heart Disease Pathways. No matter what your problem, however, my Integrative Cardiovascular Disease Prevention Program has solutions. Read on to discover how to gauge the health of your heart, find out whether you're on a Fast Track to Heart Disease or one of the earlier pathways, and what to do about it.

The Genetics Pathway:
Tests for Key Genetic Errors

Genetic errors play an important role in determining whether you wind up on one of the pathways, which one you enter, and to what extent you develop faulty arteries.

Genetic errors that cause significant problems, such as the extremely high cholesterol levels known as familial hypercholesterolemia, are easy to detect. However, many of us have relatively minor genetic changes that act subtly, predisposing us to coronary heart disease that strikes only when other factors, such as poor diet or exposure to certain chemicals, come into play.

These smaller errors are slight alterations in DNA that occur when one of the four "letters" that make up the genetic alphabet—the nucleotides known as adenine (A), cytosine (C), thymine (T), and guanine (G)—is replaced by one of the other letters. For example, perhaps the sequence of nucleotides in a segment of DNA should be ACAT—but instead, the last "letter" is changed, and the segment becomes ACAG. It's like a typo. Doctors call this a single nucleotide polymorphism (SNP).

These little "genetic typos" are common, and many are inconsequential. But suppose yours occurs within a portion of the DNA that carries instructions for the behavior of a hormone that helps regulate cholesterol. This altered hormone may not be deformed enough to trigger disease on its own, but if it is combined with other problems in the way your body handles cholesterol, it may tip the balance in favor of disease.

We know about certain genetic typos that play a role in coronary heart disease. For example, one affects the secretion of LDL and increases the risk of suffering a heart attack, while another increases the risk of coronary heart disease by interfering with one of the body's important antioxidants, leading to increased oxidative damage.

So far, more than seven hundred SNPs related to cardiovascular health, heart disease, and hypertension have been identified. Fortunately, you can be tested for SNPs that may set you on the path toward coronary heart disease at laboratories such as Pathway Genomics, Doctor's Data, Genova Diagnostics, and Quest Diagnostics. Remember, however, that these are genetic predispositions, not disasters written in stone. Knowing where you have weaknesses can be a blessing, as it allows you to take corrective action.

Chapter Two

The Integrative Cardiovascular Disease Prevention Program

I'M A TRADITIONALLY trained physician who is well versed in the use of standard medicine and surgery, but I'm also very interested in integrative, functional, and metabolic medicine (previously called complementary and alternative medicine). Over the course of my career, I've taken what I consider to be the best of both approaches to create my eight-step *Integrative Cardiovascular Disease Prevention Program*. The steps are:

1. Get thoroughly checked by a physician who goes beyond the traditional Big Five coronary heart disease risk factors to examine the biochemical variations and disease pathways I'll be discussing in the chapters to come.

2. Reduce inflammation, oxidative stress, and immune dysfunction with nutritional supplements, proper nutrition, weight loss, improvement in body composition, exercise, and medications and treat or eliminate factors that are causing or exacerbating these problems anywhere in your body. Dealing with these three problems is key, for everything else that poses a risk of coronary heart disease eventually triggers one or more of these three "late-stage" problems.

3. Counteract problems with cholesterol and blood fat; stabilize blood pressure and normalize blood flow through the

arteries; and correct abnormalities in glucose and insulin levels with optimal nutrition, exercise, weight loss, nutritional supplements, and medications. Remember that all of these problems contribute to the inflammation, oxidative stress, and immune dysfunction that damage the endothelium and set the stage for disease and possibly disaster.

4. Exercise using the ABCT (Aerobics, Build, Contour, and Tone) Exercise Program, the only one that fully taps into the muscles' ability to communicate with the rest of the body and encourage healing, slow aging of the arteries/aging in general, reduce morbidity and mortality, and promote better health.

5. Attend to any other diseases or states that may be contributing to inflammation, oxidation, autoimmune dysfunction, and/or endothelial damage or otherwise increasing the risk of coronary heart disease.

6. Make lifestyle changes to achieve ideal body weight and body composition, eliminate or reduce stress, stop smoking, sleep more, and improve your outlook on life.

7. Use standard medications as appropriate, and understand the importance of integrating scientifically proven medications with nutritional supplements.

8. Stop using *all* tobacco products.

My plan is the only one that takes into consideration all that we've learned about coronary heart disease over the past several decades, including the fact that the Big Five risk factors are not the best indicators of an impending heart attack.

The key to reducing your coronary heart disease risk is early detection, plus early and aggressive prevention and treatment of *all* identified risk predictors—in other words, everything that can damage the endothelium. It is never too late to begin. You can slow, stabilize, prevent, and even reverse coronary heart disease. My plan helps you do so by combining the best of standard functional and metabolic medicine.

In the next five chapters, we'll look at the Fast Track to Heart Disease Pathways, how and why you may find yourself on one or more of them, their dangers, plus treatments and preventive strategies.

Chapter Three

Inflammation: A Fast Track to Heart Disease

W<small>E USED TO BELIEVE</small> that "hardening of the arteries" (atherosclerosis) was triggered by excess cholesterol and fat in the bloodstream that somehow attached itself to the inner lining of an artery, like a barnacle sticks to the hull of a ship. More and more would attach, glomming on to what was already there, until sooner or later, one of these little "barnacle groups" would grow large enough to block the flow of blood. If the blockage happened to occur in an artery that fed the heart, the part of the heart that was no longer receiving fresh blood would die—in other words, a heart attack would strike. But that idea was rendered obsolete when numerous studies conducted during the past decade showed that the genesis of a heart attack involves a lot more than a clump of fat damming blood flow. We now know that one of the primary coronary heart disease risk factors is inflammation, and it plays an important role in promoting heart disease from the very beginning.

WHAT IS INFLAMMATION?

Inflammation is a natural response of the body designed to prevent infection and repair damage. You're undoubtedly familiar with the outward signs of inflammation: *swelling, redness, warmth*, and *pain*. In simple terms, here's how it works: You cut your finger, and bacteria race in through this break in the skin. Your body recognizes the bacteria as foreign invaders and undertakes to defend itself. The defense begins as the walls of nearby blood vessels "loosen up" so that plasma (the liquid part of the blood) can leak into the surrounding tissue. As the infected area floods, immune system cells in the plasma come into contact with the invading bacteria and begin to do battle. The flooding also causes swelling and creates tension in the area, triggering pain. Some red blood cells also escape from the blood vessels into the surrounding tissue, causing redness. The increased circulation of fluids promotes warmth.

All the while, the immune system cells fight with and destroy the bacteria, engaging the invaders in hand-to-hand combat, shooting out chemicals designed to destroy the enemy, literally engulfing and devouring them, and otherwise doing what it takes to protect the body. Sooner or later the battle is won, the excess fluid is reabsorbed, the immune system cells are recalled, the battlefield debris is cleared away, the pain recedes, and the body returns to normal. Mission accomplished!

This kind of inflammation is short term, beneficial, and absolutely necessary. Without it, we could not survive. But inflammation becomes a problem if it is chronic, lasting long after the initial danger has been dealt with—or perhaps arising for no reason at all. Then it serves no useful function and is very destructive to the body. With chronic inflammation, the body keeps sending out immune system soldiers after the battle has been won—or even when there has been no invasion or obvious damage. The system gets stuck in "fight mode," and the chemicals continually released by immune system cells to defend the body wind up damaging or killing the body's own cells. Thus, instead of protecting the body, the inflammatory process starts to destroy it. Chronic inflammation is believed to be the root of most degenerative diseases, including arthritis, diabetes, cancer, and heart disease.

HOW INFLAMMATION CONTRIBUTES TO CORONARY HEART DISEASE

As you recall from the discussion in chapter one, heart disease begins with a little "scratch" to the endothelium. The body repairs the injury, but during the repair process, immune system cells, oxidized LDL cholesterol, and other cells and particles can slip through the endothelium and into the artery wall, setting the stage for endothelial dysfunction and coronary heart disease.

Inflammation can start this terrible progression by causing or contributing to the initial scratch. And once the toxic brew has begun to bubble within the arterial wall, inflammation can stir the pot by serving as a beacon, drawing additional immune system cells, oxidized LDL cells, and more to the site. From start to finish, the creation and rupture of the toxic brew plaque are driven by inflammation. Among other things, inflammation:

- draws immune system cells to the injured site, where they can slip through the endothelium and into the artery wall
- alters the activity of the endothelium so that it attracts substances that contribute to the buildup of plaque
- loosens the junctions between endothelial cells, making the migration of foreign substances into the artery wall easier
- transforms helpful immune system cells called macrophages into harmful foam cells
- attracts immune system cells called T cells that, upon arrival, release substances that keep the inflammatory process going

Through these actions, the toxic brew itself becomes a source of chronic inflammation, fueling its own growth. Don't worry about the details; the key point to remember is that inflammation is present at the beginning, middle, and end of the coronary heart disease process. It is so potentially harmful that I would go so far as to say that inappropriate inflammation is much more dangerous to the artery linings than is an extra 10, 20, or even 50 cholesterol points over the ideal.

HOW TO RECOGNIZE THE SIGNS OF CHRONIC INFLAMMATION: HS-CRP

It's easy to recognize the signs of short-term inflammation: the site of the injury becomes reddened and warm, it swells, and it becomes painful. But chronic inflammation within the cardiovascular system is hidden inside the body; you can't see any overt signs of it. How do you know if it exists?

Your doctor can track inflammation and its fluctuations by measuring the levels of certain substances that rise as inflammation increases and fall as it fades away. One of the most prominent indicators of inflammation is high-sensitivity C-reactive protein (HS-CRP). This is the most predictive of all inflammation indicators, and of all the inflammatory risk factors and mediators, HS-CRP is backed by the best scientific research. It should be part of every blood exam done for patients. Levels over 2.0 mg/L are cause for concern.

Many things can increase levels of HS-CRP, which is a protein produced by the liver from substances such as interleukin-6 (IL-6), interleukin-1B, and tumor necrosis factor alpha (TNF-alpha). These and other inflammatory markers and substances from all over the body travel to the liver, where they are processed into HS-CRP.

Any infection will trigger an increase in HS-CRP, including periodontal disease, *H. pylori* infection, a sore throat, streptococcal infection, pneumonia, colitis, and sinusitis. Any acute injury that damages tissue will also trigger inflammation and increase HS-CRP. If there's no obvious reason for a rising HS-CRP—such as a sore throat or an injury—the increase is probably due to inflammation within the arterial system. Although HS-CRP is not itself an infection, it acts in many ways to promote inflammation as well as the oxidative stress and autoimmune dysfunction that harm the endothelium.

HS-CRP is thus both a risk factor and a risk mediator for coronary heart disease. In other words, it predicts an increased risk for heart disease, but it also causes continued damage to the arteries as long as it is elevated. For these reasons, HS-CRP should be checked at regular intervals, which can be done with a simple blood test. And if it is elevated, no matter what the reason, it is very important to reduce it to normal levels as rapidly as possible to avoid damage to the arteries.

Sometimes, the underlying cause of the elevation is a disease that can be identified and treated. For example, a 2010 study published in the journal *Angiology* reported that otherwise healthy adults with chronic periodontal disease had significantly higher levels of HS-CRP and interleukin-6 compared with a control group that did not have the disease. But when the periodontal disease was treated, the levels of these inflammation markers fell significantly.[1] I've seen elevated HS-CRP in patients with a variety of diseases, including a middle-aged man suffering from severe osteoarthritis and obesity whose HS-CRP dropped from 8 to 1 mg/L when both were treated and a young woman whose HS-CRP fell from an alarming 22 to a very safe level of 2 mg/L when her chronic bronchitis was eliminated by antibiotics. In another patient with *H. pylori* infection, which was causing his stomach ulcers, HS-CRP dropped from 6 to 1.5 mg/L with antibiotic treatment.

In a great many cases, however, the HS-CRP elevation is

due to long-term lifestyle and dietary factors. This may sound like bad news, but it's actually good, for it means you can start making helpful changes today—and the diet and exercise regimen I discuss later will help you do so.

I urge you to have your HS-CRP checked as soon as possible to see if you are harboring inflammation that may be damaging your arteries. Your physician may want to order other tests to search for inflammation or to provide more information about the inflammation. These include tests for serum amyloid A, which is secreted in the body during the acute phase of inflammation; IL-6, which is a small molecule that promotes the immune response; TNF-alpha, which plays a role in the acute stage of the inflammatory process and the production of HS-CRP; neopterin, a substance produced by macrophages that both shows inflammation is present and may increase atherosclerosis; and uric acid, high levels of which induce arterial inflammation. Having elevated levels of any one of these or other inflammation markers is like walking on those little Variations Pathways in the Heart Disease Maze.

In addition, get yourself checked for chronic periodontal infection and other "quiet" infections that may have been festering in your body for some time, as well as for increased levels of heavy metals such as mercury, lead, arsenic, cadmium, and iron in your bloodstream and body tissues. These substances increase inflammation (and oxidative stress), damaging the arteries and leading to coronary heart disease.

THE "UNMEASURABLE" INDICATORS

The inflammation indicators I just mentioned can all be measured and quantified, but there are some others that can't. These are items or situations that are likely to contribute to inflammation, but we can't say that X amount of one of these leads to a 3-percent increase in inflammation or anything similar.

However, we can say with certainty that the risk of inflammation rises with any of the following conditions:

- increased intake of refined carbohydrates, including sugars and sweets
- increased intake of trans-fatty acids and saturated fats
- smoking
- lack of sleep
- lack of exercise
- *H. pylori* and other chronic infections
- chronic autoimmune and inflammatory diseases, such as rheumatoid arthritis, chronic obstructive pulmonary disease, and lupus

NATURAL WAYS TO SLOW OR REVERSE CHRONIC INFLAMMATION

I urge you to get tested for HS-CRP and other inflammation indicators. If the tests indicate that your body is in an inflamed state, the time to do something about it is now.

Knowing that inflammation is a major culprit in heart disease, you may wonder if you can simply eradicate it, just as you might destroy the bacteria that's causing an infection in your finger. That would be a bad thing. Remember, short-term inflammation is absolutely necessary as a part of the body's natural defenses. Without it, you would die. What you really want to do is prevent the ongoing inflammation that serves no useful purpose.

Your doctor can prescribe various medicines that will help quell unnecessary inflammation. These are sometimes necessary, but like all drugs, they can trigger side effects. That's why I like to begin with natural means of reducing inflammation when possible—like giving up all tobacco products and losing excess body fat, especially abdominal fat. There are also a number of foods, food components, and supplements that have anti-inflammatory properties. They include the following items:

- *Arginine*—This naturally occurring amino acid has been shown to lower homocysteine levels and blood pressure, two factors that increase inflammation. (We'll talk more about homocysteine in Appendix II.)
- *Boswellia*—An herbal extract derived from the *Boswellia* tree and used in ayurvedic medicine, it helps block a pro-inflammatory enzyme called 5-LOX that strongly promotes atherosclerosis.
- *Carnosine*—A peptide present in the heart, skeletal muscle, and other parts of the body that helps reduce inflammation (as well as oxidation).
- *Coenzyme Q10 (CoQ10)*—Naturally produced by the body, CoQ10 participates in a number of reactions and has anti-inflammatory properties, inhibiting proinflammatory substances such as TNF-alpha.[2] Animal studies have shown that supplementation with CoQ10 enhances the anti-inflammatory properties of vitamin E.[3]
- *Curcumin*—Also known as turmeric, curcumin contains substances called curcuminoids that have anti-inflammatory properties.
- *Flavonoids*—This large class of plant chemicals (phytochemicals) is found in fruits and vegetables, especially those with colorful skins, and includes such substances as genistein, hesperidin, rutin, and the catechins. The flavonoids are potent inflammation fighters due in part to their modulation of certain proinflammatory genes. They have also been shown to reduce the number of arterial scratches, strengthen blood vessel walls, and deactivate free radicals.
- *Gamma-linolenic acid (GLA)*—An omega-6 fatty acid found in black currant seed oil, borage oil, and evening

primrose oil, GLA boosts levels of prostaglandin E_1, which suppresses inflammation.

- *Ginseng*—A well-known Asian plant, ginseng contains ginsenosides, biologically active compounds that have anti-inflammatory effects.
- *Lutein*—A nutrient found in spinach and other dark-green, leafy vegetables, lutein is best known for its ability to protect against macular degeneration through its anti-inflammatory actions. Higher blood levels of lutein have also been associated with lower levels of the important inflammation marker C-reactive protein.
- *Lycopene*—A red pigment found in tomatoes and tomato products, lycopene is known for its antioxidant effects and its ability to fight inflammation. One study found that drinking tomato juice lowered levels of TNF-alpha, an inflammation marker, by nearly 35 percent. Lycopene may also help reduce the inflammation associated with obesity by interfering with the production of proinflammatory substances in adipose tissue.
- *Omega-3 fatty acids*—The omega-3 fatty acids, found in cold-water fatty fish such as cod, tuna, mackerel, salmon, herring, and anchovies, form the basis of many of the body's natural anti-inflammatory compounds. The main dietary omega-3s are eicosapentaenoic acid (EPA) and docosahexaenoic acid (DHA).
- *R-lipoic acid*—A superior antioxidant, r-lipoic acid is the form of alpha-lipoic acid (ALA) that occurs in plants, animals, and the human body. However, it is ten times more effective than ALA, significantly reducing inflammation while increasing or maintaining levels of other important antioxidants, including vitamins C and E and glutathione.
- *Vitamin C, vitamin E, and selenium*—These antioxidants quell the free radical damage that contributes to inflammation.

- *Vitamin D*—Often referred to as the "sunshine vitamin," vitamin D is well known for its role in maintaining strong bones and teeth. However, it also has anti-inflammatory properties, lowering both C-reactive protein (CRP) and IL-6.
- *Vitamin K*—The form of vitamin K known as vitamin K_2 (MK7), found in supplement form, reduces inflammation by lowering IL-6 levels. It may also reverse the accumulation of coronary artery plaque.
- *Zinc*—This anti-inflammatory mineral is believed to work by decreasing inflammation-producing compounds called cytokines.

RECOMMENDATIONS

The list of supplements above may be overwhelming, but don't worry; you don't have to take all of them. (In fact, you shouldn't.) I have just listed them here to show you the wide array of natural anti-inflammatory substances available.

I highly recommend that you begin with the following daily regimen, adding a few of the supplements listed above if you wish. After a period of three months or so, get your blood levels of inflammation markers rechecked to see if they have improved. If not, you and your physician should consider selecting additional antioxidant supplements to add to your basic daily regimen.

Daily Regimen

1. An Anti-inflammatory Diet

An anti-inflammatory diet is high in omega-3 fatty acids and monounsaturated fatty acids (e.g., olive oil); low in saturated fat, trans fats, and fried foods; high in fresh fruits and vegetables; and very low in refined carbohydrates. (See chapter nine for a complete discussion of diet for heart disease prevention and my Integrative Cardiovascular Disease Prevention Program Diet.)

2. Exercise

Regular exercise has been shown to reduce levels of the inflammation marker HS-CRP. In one study, Greek researchers followed sixty overweight diabetics, some of whom were assigned to a six-month-long aerobic exercise program and some of whom did not exercise.[4] Among the exercisers, average HS-CRP fell by half, while their interleukin-18 (a cytokine able to induce severe inflammatory reactions) levels dropped by one-third. The researchers noted that aerobic exercise "exerts anti-inflammatory effects" in people with type 2 diabetes, even if they don't lose weight while exercising. Other studies have found that resistance training with weights, rather than aerobic exercise, is the key to reducing HS-CRP. In one such study, resistance exercise caused HS-CRP to fall by 32.8 percent, compared with a 16.1-percent fall with aerobic exercise.[5] Since a good exercise program should include both aerobic and resistance exercises, as well as stretching, you'll enjoy the inflammation-lowering benefits from both types. (See chapter ten for a complete discussion of exercise for heart disease prevention.)

3. Omega-3 Fatty Acid Supplement Containing EPA and DHA: 3 to 4 grams of EPA and DHA combined, in a 3:2 ratio

Numerous studies have shown that there is an inverse relationship between omega-3 consumption and inflammation, with HS-CRP levels falling as omega-3 levels rise. In a recent study, Japanese researchers examined the diets and HS-CRP levels of 443 young Japanese women, ages eighteen to twenty-two.[6] The consumption of omega-3 fatty acids was found to be inversely associated with HS-CRP levels; that is, the more omega-3s in their blood, the lower their HS-CRP levels.

4. Gamma-Linolenic Acid (GLA): 1.5 to 2 grams

GLA fights inflammation by increasing levels of the anti-inflammatory compound prostaglandin E1. It works synergistically with omega-3s.

5. Vitamin C: 500 grams twice daily

Vitamin C has been shown to significantly lower levels of HS-CRP. Researchers from the University of California at Berkeley tested the effects of 1,000 milligrams vitamin C per day for two months in healthy nonsmokers.[7] They found that among those with CRP high enough to put them at risk of developing cardiovascular disease, vitamin C reduced CRP levels by an average of 25 percent, which was comparable to the inflammation-reducing effects of taking a statin drug.

6. Vitamin E: 400 to 800 international units in the gamma-/delta-tocopherol form as well as some tocotrienols

Vitamin E is a major antioxidant that helps fight the free radical damage that causes endothelial dysfunction. Vitamin E in the gamma-/delta-tocopherol and tocotrienol forms has been shown to significantly lower both HS-CRP and interleukin-6.

A MAJOR PROBLEM WHEN IT'S OUT OF WHACK

Remember, inflammation is a significant cause of the "scratches" that set the stage for heart disease, and the inflammation response to these wounds can quickly become chronic. Eventually, the build-up of inflammatory substances, toxins, and clotting factors can explode into the bloodstream, producing a clot and triggering a heart attack. Although inflammation is a natural process, it is often triggered inappropriately or continues well past the helpful point, which then makes it harmful. Inflammation is a significant cause of coronary heart disease and a much more serious threat than just about any other indicator of impending heart disease.

If your inflammation levels are even slightly high, do whatever it takes to bring them down to safe levels.

Chapter Four

Quenching Oxidation, a Disaster in the Making

Everybody has heard of antioxidants, most notably vitamins C and E, and knows that they help to combat something bad. But you may have found yourself wondering what exactly the antioxidants are combating. It sounds like oxygen, but doesn't the body need oxygen?

Oxygen is necessary to the energy-producing processes of the cell, and without it we would die. Yet endlessly interacting with oxygen also stresses the body. The problem is oxidation, a natural biochemical process that occurs constantly and results in the production of highly reactive molecules called free radicals, unbalanced molecules that interact with other molecules within the cell, causing damage to proteins, cell membranes, and genes.

The damage occurs when a free radical "steals" an electron from another molecule in an attempt to balance itself, leaving the second molecule unbalanced and unable to function properly. To rebalance itself, the second molecule might aggressively snatch an electron from a third molecule, damaging that molecule in the process. If it can't find another electron, it will either die or continue to function in an altered way that harms the body. Needless to say, if this chain of electron stealing goes on too long and too many healthy molecules are affected, widespread damage can ensue, not only to molecules but to cells, tissues, organs, and even entire bodily systems. Although the term oxidation *can* refer to the combining of oxygen with another substance—say, oxygen plus carbon equals carbon dioxide (CO_2)—it is usually used to refer to the process in which a molecule loses one or more electrons while interacting with another molecule, regardless of whether oxygen is involved.

Like inflammation, oxidation is a biochemical reaction necessary to life that causes problems only when it gets out of hand—when it happens too often or when the wrong substances are oxidized. Uncontrolled oxidation and free radical production contribute to and worsen many conditions, including heart disease, macular degeneration, diabetes, and cancer. They are also thought to be a major cause of aging.

Some Diseases/Conditions Related to Oxidative Stress

- Aging
- Alzheimer's disease
- Arthritis
- Atherosclerosis (coronary heart disease)
- Cancer
- Cataracts
- Diabetes
- Emphysema
- Heart attack
- Inflammatory bowel disease
- Kidney disease
- Macular degeneration
- Multiple sclerosis
- Pancreatitis
- Parkinson's disease
- Skin lesions
- Stroke

DEFENDING AGAINST OXIDATION

To keep the electron stealing under control and to ward off excessive amounts of free radical damage, the body produces substances called antioxidants and takes in additional antioxidants through the diet. One way the antioxidants help is by acting as electron donors to rebalance free radicals. That is, they supply the missing electron to an unbalanced molecule, so it doesn't need to steal another one from some other molecule. The body's primary antioxidants are glutathione peroxidase (GP), catalase, and superoxide dismutase (SOD), while the major antioxidants that come from foods include vitamins (vitamin E, vitamin C), carotenoids (beta-carotene, lycopene), flavonoids, and polyphenols (from herbs, teas, and grape skin).

When there aren't enough antioxidants available to the body to neutralize its load of free radicals, the body is said to be in *oxidative stress*. The result is minor to massive cell damage that can cause cellular mutations, tissue breakdown, and a compromised immune system.

HOW OXIDATIVE STRESS CONTRIBUTES TO HEART DISEASE

Oxidative stress/free radical damage plays a crucial part in initiating and promoting heart disease, primarily through its effect on LDL cholesterol. Like HDL, LDL contains lipids that can be oxidized. But HDL has a built-in advantage: an enzyme called paraoxonase (PON), which helps ward off oxidation. Unfortunately, the LDL molecule has no such protection, so it is more likely to become oxidized. In its normal state, LDL doesn't contribute to heart disease. It doesn't become dangerous until it is attacked by free radicals and oxidized. Then, LDL turns "sticky" and is much more likely to cling to artery walls. It also becomes an irritant that can cause the microscopic "scratch" on the artery wall that starts the buildup of plaque and the formation of the toxic brew.

From that point on, oxidized LDL continues to play a role in virtually all stages of coronary heart disease. It causes inflammatory cells such as macrophages and blood-clotting factors such as platelets to rush to the injured spot and stick to the artery wall. It spurs the conversion of monocytes into foam cells, promotes the development of fatty streaks, and encourages the accumulation of cells and other substances that make up the toxic brew.

Oxidized LDL is so wrapped up in the coronary heart disease process that measuring its blood levels is a very accurate method of distinguishing between those who have coronary heart disease and those who don't. But oxidized LDL isn't the only villain in the oxidation–heart disease story. Uncontrolled free radical activity is also linked to activation of the metallomatrix proteins (MMPs), which can wear away at the fibrous cap on an arterial plaque and lead to the spewing of its toxic brew. Oxidation is also intimately connected to inflammation, with one egging on the other. Oxidation causes damage to cells and tissues, spurring inflammation. And the inflammatory process produces additional free radicals, which can further damage tissues. It's a vicious circle.

In short, oxidation is a necessary, inevitable process that, when uncontrolled, causes severe damage to bodily tissues, organs, and systems, including and especially the cardiovascular system. It further exacerbates the problem by encouraging inflammation, which promotes greater amounts of oxidative stress.

WHAT CAUSES OXIDATIVE STRESS?

Diet is a major source of oxidative stress. We eat foods that have undergone oxidation (think of apple slices that have turned brown) and consume oils that oxidize when they become even slightly rancid. When foods are fried at high temperatures, the bonds in the molecules that make up the foods can become unstable, producing free radicals. Smoked, barbecued, and charbroiled foods also contain substances that either become oxidized or encourage the oxidation of other substances once they enter the body. The dietary factors that contribute to an increase in oxidative stress include the following:

- *Reduced Intake of Antioxidants*—An insufficient intake of antioxidants (in food or supplement form) lowers the number of "troops" the body can send out to quell free radicals, allowing oxidative processes to dominate.
- *Increased Intake of Refined Carbohydrates, Including Sugar and Sweets*—These foods cause a rapid rise in blood glucose that promotes inflammation and oxidative stress, even when after-meal glucose levels are in the normal range.
- *Increased Intake of Dietary Fats*—A high intake of fat, especially saturated fat, significantly increases the number of free radicals in the body, damaging artery linings and possibly causing artery spasms.
- *Increased Intake of Trans-Fatty Acids*—These "fake" fats, which include hydrogenated and partially hydrogenated fats, are often found in margarine, shortening, and commercially prepared baked and fried foods. Studies have shown that these substances are potent generators of free radicals that damage the cardiovascular system.

Other factors that increase oxidative stress include the following:

- *Elevated Levels of Iron and Ferritin in the Blood*—Too much iron or ferritin (a form of iron) increases inflammation and free radical production. This damages the artery linings, setting the stage for coronary heart disease, especially in men.

- *Increased Levels of Heavy Metals in Blood and Tissue*—Like iron and ferritin, elevated levels of mercury, lead, cadmium, and other heavy metals increase free radical production and inflammation, damaging the linings of the arteries and promoting cardiovascular disease.
- *Myeloperoxidase*—This enzyme made from white blood cells oxidizes HDL cholesterol and apolipoprotein A, making these substances unable to protect the arteries against oxidation and damage from LDL cholesterol.
- *Excessive Stress*—As emotional stress increases, so does free radical production. If the stress is mild to moderate, the body can usually handle the increased oxidation. But if it's excessive, free radicals can overwhelm the body's immune system.
- *Obesity*—An excess of fatty tissue, especially if it is found in the abdominal area, is directly linked to high HS-CRP levels, an indication of both increased oxidation and inflammation.
- *Cigarette Smoke*—Cigarette smoke produces tremendous amounts of free radicals—even secondhand smoke. While antioxidants can decrease oxidative stress in smokers, they cannot eliminate it.
- *Sunlight*—Exposure to the UVA and UVB rays in sunlight produces large amounts of free radicals within the skin.
- *Radiation Therapy and Chemotherapy*—These two treatments cause a tremendous increase in free radical production and lead to oxidative stress, no matter which part of the body is involved.

Additional sources of oxidative stress include environmental pollutants, toxins, certain medications, excessive exercise, alcohol, and many illnesses, including depression.

HOW TO RECOGNIZE OXIDATIVE STRESS

How do you determine if your body is handling its free radical load adequately and is steering clear of oxidative stress? Several tests can indicate excessive levels of oxidative stress and/or weakened oxidative defenses by measuring the by-products of oxidation or damage to the cells. High-sensitivity C-reactive protein (HS-CRP) is a useful indicator of oxidation. You'll remember from the previous chapter that HS-CRP is normally thought of as an indicator of inflammation, not oxidation, but an intricate relationship exists between oxidative stress and inflammation. Oxidative stress may be a determinant of HS-CRP, so measuring HS-CRP levels can be another way of gauging it. Levels over 2.0 mg/L may indicate oxidative stress.

There are other helpful tests, including ones for 8-hydroxyguanosine (8-OHG) and 8-hydroxy-2'-deoxyguanosine (8-OHdG), which are by-products of oxidized DNA and RNA, and for malondialdehyde (MDA), which is a by-product of lipid peroxidation. The comet assay quantifies and analyzes DNA damage in individual cells. Measuring thiobarbituric acid reactive substances (TBARS) checks lipid peroxidation levels, and measuring 8-isoprostane identifies a compound formed from the free radical–driven peroxidation of essential fatty acids.

In addition, you can measure the levels of various antioxidant molecules that, when in short supply, render the body less able to handle oxidants and more likely to be in a state of oxidative stress. Some common ones include glutathione, superoxide dismutase (SOD), and catalase.

Your physician can help you decide which test(s) you should undergo, and you certainly don't need all of them. For my patients, I usually order HS-CRP, and if the results show signs of excessive oxidative stress, I may follow up with the MDA and 8-OHdG tests to confirm.

ANTIOXIDANTS—A KEY TO CONTROLLING OXIDATIVE STRESS

Studies of large population groups make it clear that low blood levels of antioxidants are associated with an increased risk of developing coronary heart disease. Conversely, high levels of antioxidants reduce the risk of heart disease, strokes, and other diseases of the cardiovascular system.

Researchers used to think an antioxidant-rich diet protected against diseases related to oxidative stress by supplying enough donor electrons to quell free radicals and prevent future damage. And while the strategy *is* effective, the rationale behind it doesn't quite make sense. That's because the antioxidants obtainable from foods or supplements don't contain enough donor electrons to quell the massive numbers of free radicals harbored by the body. This puzzling state of affairs led most researchers to suspect that antioxidants work against oxidation in more ways than one—a theory that has turned out to be true. When it comes to heart disease, antioxidants supply several protective and beneficial effects that go above and beyond simply donating electrons. For example:

- They make it more difficult for substances to stick to artery walls by inhibiting cellular adhesion molecules.
- They slow the release of proinflammatory substances called cytokines, which lessens inflammation and the production of excessive free radicals.
- They discourage the formation of unwanted blood clots, lessening the chances of blockages.
- They positively affect the "nutrient-genetic" interaction, turning on good genes that reduce oxidative stress, inflammation, and immune dysfunction; improve cell health; and reduce heart disease. They also turn off bad genes that increase oxidative stress, inflammation, and

immune dysfunction and cause cell dysfunction and heart disease.

Individual antioxidants confer special protection. For example, various tocopherols (forms of vitamin E) can fight inflammation by boosting nitric oxide and lowering HS-CRP and IL-6, improve endothelial dysfunction, and encourage the relaxation of arterial muscles to lower blood pressure and accommodate blood flow.

Vitamin C works its own wonders. Like vitamin E, it improves endothelial dysfunction and helps lower blood pressure. But it can also increase arterial elasticity—the ability to "expand" as necessary—and reduce HS-CRP. Through various pathways and mechanisms, antioxidants help your body fight the deleterious effects of oxidation.

Sources of Antioxidants

Your antioxidant supply comes from three sources: internal manufacture, foods, and supplements.

Antioxidants That Occur Naturally in the Body

Our bodies produce some of the strongest, most effective antioxidants in existence. These substances are absolutely critical to the effective function of the immune system and to the preservation of health. The primary antioxidants manufactured by the body include

- *Alpha-Lipoic Acid (ALA)*—This fatty antioxidant is used to convert blood sugar into energy. Because it can function in both water and fat, it acts in more areas of the body than most antioxidants. It also helps "deoxidize" oxidized LDL and recharges vitamin C and other antioxidants that have been "used up" after a single antioxidation battle.

Unfortunately, the body's ability to produce ALA declines with age, which is why many people begin to run low in their forties and fifties. When used as a supplement, the preferred form is r-lipoic acid (RLA), as this is the form used by the cell mitochondria.

- *Coenzyme Q10 (CoQ10)*—This natural substance assists in many reactions, including the extraction of energy from food. It serves as an antioxidant and protects LDL from oxidation. In addition, CoQ10 lowers blood pressure, improves heart function, and combats coronary heart disease, angina, chronic heart failure, and others. CoQ10 levels typically begin to fall at about age thirty, and a great many people have moderately or severely low levels.

- *Glutathione*—This is the most abundant antioxidant in the body, commonly called "the master antioxidant." A lack of glutathione has been associated with increased free radical and oxidative damage. Glutathione guards against coronary heart disease and heart attack, lowers blood pressure, improves immune function, decreases inflammation, and slows vascular aging.

- *Melatonin*—A hormone produced in the brain that helps regulate sleep cycles, melatonin lowers oxidative stress, inflammation, and blood pressure, and improves endothelial dysfunction. In addition to being manufactured by the body, melatonin is found in vegetables, fruits, grains, and herbs.

Antioxidant Highlight: Glutathione

Glutathione has several duties in the body, including aiding in the synthesis of DNA and strengthening the immune system. But it is best known as an antioxidant that protects cells from the free radical called hydrogen peroxide. It also slows the oxidation of fats, helps other antioxidants do their job, and can reduce both blood pressure and the risk of heart attack. One study looked at 636 people with suspected coronary heart disease, dividing them into four groups, depending on their levels of red blood cell glutathione.[1] Those in the quarter with the highest levels of glutathione had a 71 percent lower risk of heart attack compared with those in the lowest quarter.

Unfortunately, glutathione production begins to decline at around age twenty, leaving many people older than that with a major breach in their antioxidant defenses. Taking the mineral selenium can help, as it is necessary for production of the antioxidant, and low selenium levels can impair its activity. Glutathione levels can be increased by taking special liposomal forms of glutathione orally or by taking certain glutathione precursors, including RLA, n-acetyl cysteine (NAC), and whey protein.

Unfortunately, due to the natural decline in production and other issues, most people can't rely solely on the body's naturally occurring antioxidants. They also need to take in sufficient amounts of antioxidants from the outside, preferably through foods and food components.

Antioxidants from Foods and Food Components

Fruits and vegetables are excellent sources of antioxidants. They provide antioxidants in combination rather than singly, which can increase their beneficial effects and confer additional protection.

Back in 1997, French researchers reported that increasing the intake of fruits and vegetables until they provided 30 milligrams of antioxidant carotenoids made LDL less susceptible to oxidization after only two weeks.[2] Similarly, a study utilizing volunteers in Ireland, Spain, France, and the Netherlands found that "increased consumption of carotenoid-rich fruits and vegetables did increase LDL oxidation resistance."[3]

Another study looked at eighteen healthy adults who consumed their normal diets and took fish oil supplements for three weeks, added five portions of fruits and vegetables for the next three weeks, then returned to their normal diets again for the final three weeks.[4] During the time they were eating the extra fruits and vegetables, their blood levels of the antioxidants vitamin C, lutein, beta-cryptoxanthin, alpha-carotene, and beta-carotene increased significantly. There was a reduction in the susceptibility of LDL to oxidation. In one of my own studies, a high dose of a fruit and vegetable extract not only reduced blood pressure but also slowed the progression of coronary heart disease in the coronary arteries.[5]

The Lyon Diet Heart Study found that adopting the Mediterranean-style diet, based on vegetables and other foods rich in natural antioxidants, leads to a reduction in risk of coronary heart disease or related illnesses. And here's the fascinating part: sometimes the heart disease risk drops with the Mediterranean diet *even though cholesterol and blood fat levels remain about the same!* This is undoubtedly due to the decrease in oxidative stress and inflammation brought about by the diet's high antioxidant content and its ability to reduce inflammation. This emphasizes the point I've been making about cholesterol being just one element in the heart disease equation—often a less important factor than oxidation and inflammation.

Best Food Sources of Antioxidants

According to a U.S. Department of Agriculture study that tested more than one hundred foods, the twenty fruits, vegetables, and nuts that contain the most antioxidants are as follows:

1. Small red bean (dried), ½ cup
2. Wild blueberry, 1 cup
3. Red kidney bean (dried), ½ cup
4. Pinto bean, ½ cup
5. Blueberry (cultivated), 1 cup
6. Cranberry, 1 cup (whole)
7. Artichoke (cooked hearts), 1 cup
8. Blackberry, 1 cup
9. Prune, ½ cup
10. Raspberry, 1 cup
11. Strawberry, 1 cup
12. Red Delicious apple, 1
13. Granny Smith apple, 1
14. Pecan, 1 ounce
15. Sweet cherry, 1 cup
16. Black plum, 1
17. Russet potato, 1 cooked
18. Black bean (dried), ½ cup
19. Plum, 1
20. Gala apple, 1

Certain components of food have been found to have particularly strong antioxidant effects. They include the following substances:

- *Curcumin*—This substance found in the spice turmeric inhibits the activity of enzymes that encourage inflammation within the body (such as cyclooxygenase-2 and lipoxygenase). It also reduces oxidized LDL.
- *Flavonoids*—A large group of compounds with antioxidant and other health-protective effects found in vegetables, fruits, tea, coffee, wine, and fruit juice. In addition to other actions, they reduce blood pressure.
- *Allicin*—A strong antioxidant found in garlic, allicin decreases oxidized LDL, reduces inflammation, and lowers blood pressure.
- *Lutein*—A member of the carotenoid family and therefore related to vitamin A and beta-carotene, lutein lowers oxidized LDL and blood pressure. It's found in egg yolks, dark-green leafy vegetables, tomatoes, carrots, corn, and other fruits and vegetables that contain red, orange, or yellow pigments.
- *Lycopene*—A pigment that imparts a red color to watermelon, tomatoes, and other fruits and vegetables, this member of the carotenoid family is an antioxidant, lowers blood pressure, and decreases endothelial dysfunction.
- *Resveratrol*—A substance found in grapes, purple grape juice, red wine, peanuts, and some berries. Resveratrol helps protect the arteries, improves endothelial dysfunction and arterial elasticity, inhibits blood clots, lowers cholesterol and oxidized LDL, reduces the uptake of oxidized LDL by macrophages, lowers glucose and blood pressure, and slows aging in animals. It also helps reduce weight and body fat.
- *Whey Protein*—Found in the liquid that remains after milk has been curdled and strained, whey protein contains peptides that serve as precursors to glutathione. It also lowers blood pressure and improves exercise ability and lean muscle mass.

Antioxidant Highlight: Green Tea

Green tea is a good source of antioxidants thanks to its catechins, a particular kind of flavonoid found almost exclusively in this kind of tea. The catechins, especially one named epigallocatechin gallate (EGCG), are well known for their heart-protective effects, including the lowering of cholesterol, inhibition of platelet clumping, and protection of LDL against oxidation. In a 2006 study conducted in Portugal, thirty-four volunteers drank eleven cups of water per day for three weeks, then switched to eleven cups of green tea per day for four weeks.[6] Before and after the four weeks devoted to green tea, the researchers measured the volunteers' total antioxidant status and other indicators of oxidative stress. They found that drinking green tea reduced the development of or increase in oxidative stress.

British researchers tested the antioxidant effects of green tea in a group of sixteen volunteers who were randomly assigned to one of two groups.[7] Group 1 consumed a standardized diet for three weeks, then switched to the same diet plus a green tea extract, while Group 2 began with the standardized diet plus green tea extract, then switched to the diet without green tea. While the volunteers were taking the green tea extract, their plasma antioxidant capacity (ability to combat oxidation) was higher. But the effect was short-lived, with the increase falling soon after they stopped taking the green tea extract. This suggests that green tea must be taken regularly to produce ongoing, long-term benefits.

Antioxidants from Supplements

While antioxidants function best when found in the combinations that occur naturally in foods, they can also be effective in supplement form. Some of the most common antioxidants found in supplement form include the following:

- *Beta-Carotene*—The plant form of vitamin A found in carrots, pumpkin, squash, and other orange or yellow-orange foods, as well as in broccoli, spinach, and other dark-green leafy vegetables.
- *Niacin (Vitamin B$_3$)*—A member of the B family of vitamins found in chicken, turkey, beef, salmon, peaches, bulgur wheat, and other foods. Niacin functions as a potent antioxidant, lowering oxidized LDL, VLDL, lipoprotein(a), and triglycerides; increasing helpful HDL-2 and apolipoprotein A-I; lessening oxidative stress and inflammation; and much more.
- *Selenium*—A mineral found in poultry, meat, fish, and whole grains, and in smaller amounts in fruits and vegetables. Selenium guards against oxidation by serving as part of the enzyme glutathione peroxidase. It also reduces the risk of coronary heart disease and heart attack.
- *Vitamin C*—An antioxidant found in fresh fruits and vegetables, including guava, papaya, red peppers, cantaloupe, kiwi, and orange. The vitamin "rearms" vitamin E and glutathione, allowing them to remain in the fight against free radicals longer. It also improves endothelial dysfunction and the ability of the arteries to stretch and contract on demand, which improves blood pressure.
- *Vitamin E*—A group of related substances, known as the tocopherols and tocotrienols, that have the ability to "deoxidize" oxidized LDL and improve endothelial dysfunction.

Vitamin E is found in green leafy vegetables, broccoli, brussels sprouts, nuts, seeds, and green beans. In supplement form, vitamin E is most effective in the form gamma-/delta-tocotrienols.

- *Zinc*—This mineral's most noted antioxidant effects take place in the eye, where it protects against the macular damage that can lead to blindness. Zinc is found in meat, eggs, and seafood, with smaller amounts in peas, beans, lentils, and whole grains.

In the Recommendations section below, I've included a few of what I believe are the most important and effective supplements. In chapter nine, I'll describe the Integrative Cardiovascular Disease Prevention Program Diet, a plan that will help ensure that you'll get plenty of antioxidants in their most absorbable and useful forms on a daily basis.

RECOMMENDATIONS

As you can see, there are a great many ways to combat oxidative stress—and some of them are quite delicious! I suggest that you read chapter nine immediately to learn how to put together and consume a diet that's loaded with antioxidants. Then follow the daily regimen I have outlined below. Consuming plenty of antioxidants in the form of whole foods may be the single most important way to boost the health of your heart (and the rest of your body). Get the whole family to eat this way, and see how healthy all of you can become.

Daily Regimen

By following these suggestions, you will do much to help your body combat oxidation, increase its oxidative defenses, decrease atherosclerosis, and ward off coronary heart disease.

1. Antioxidant-Rich Diet

An anti-inflammatory diet is high in omega-3 fatty acids and monounsaturated fatty acids (e.g., olive oil); low in saturated fat, trans fats, and fried foods; high in fresh fruits and vegetables; and very low in refined carbohydrates. (See chapter nine for a complete discussion of diet for heart disease prevention and a description of my Integrative Cardiovascular Disease Prevention Program Diet.)

2. Regular Exercise

(See chapter ten for a complete discussion of exercise for heart disease prevention.)

3. Coenzyme Q10: 100 to 200 milligrams per day

CoQ10 has antioxidant properties, protects LDL from oxidation, reduces lipoprotein(a) levels, and improves endothelial dysfunction. Taking statin medications such as Lipitor (atorvastatin) can cause the body to run short of CoQ10. For this reason, everyone taking a statin medicine should consider taking CoQ10 supplements. Even those who do not take statins should take CoQ10, as it helps to quell both inflammation and oxidation. Either use a highly absorbable form that says "nano" or "combined with liposome or fat delivery system" on the label, or take CoQ10 with small amounts of fatty foods to increase absorption.

4. Epigallocatechin Gallate (EGCG): 500 milligrams twice per day

The strongest health-promoting component in green tea, EGCG inhibits LDL oxidation and protects cells from lipid peroxidation and free radical damage to DNA. It has also been shown to have other heart-protective effects, including the lowering of total and LDL cholesterol, a reduction in blood pressure, and anti-inflammatory actions.

5. Resveratrol: 250 milligrams per day in the trans-resveratrol form

Resveratrol is a powerful antioxidant found in the skin of grapes, purple grape juice, red wine, peanuts, and some berries. It protects against the oxidation of both LDL and HDL, reduces atherosclerosis (in animals), and helps slow the aging of the arteries. Only use the "trans" form, as this is the most easily absorbed.

6. Vitamin C: 200 to 500 milligrams per day

Perhaps the best known antioxidant, vitamin C works together with vitamin E, "recycling" it and quenching the free radicals that result from the metabolism of vitamin E. Studies of large populations show that the risk of coronary heart disease decreases as vitamin C consumption increases. Its heart-healthy actions include combating oxidation and lowering levels of total cholesterol, LDL, and triglycerides while increasing HDL, improving endothelial dysfunction, and reducing the formation of blood clots.

7. Vitamin E: 400 milligrams per day in the form of gamma-/delta-tocotrienols

Vitamin E is a major antioxidant that helps fight the free radical damage that results in oxidized LDL and endothelial dysfunction. Because it is fat soluble, it can get through cell membranes and help fight free radical damage that might otherwise penetrate the cell's protective covering. The gamma-/delta-tocotrienol form is most effective.

Reduce Stress

When you are under severe emotional stress, your free radical production increases exponentially and can throw your body into severe oxidative stress. Hormones released during stressful times—such as cortisol and catecholamines—break down into powerful free radicals capable of wreaking havoc on the body. Practice some form of concerted relaxation every day, if possible. Do yoga, meditate, or take a warm bath while listening to soothing music. Destressing is a vitally important part of any health program and an excellent way to reduce your level of oxidative stress.

Defanging Oxidation

As long as you continue to breathe, the erosive process of oxidation will continue in your body. It's inevitable, but you can do much in the way of damage control by consuming plenty of antioxidants, exercising, and reducing your stress level.

Chapter Five

Fixing Cholesterol: Beyond the Numbers

ELEVATED CHOLESTEROL IS *not* the boogeyman we've been told it is, and having elevated levels of total and LDL cholesterol does *not* mean that you're all but guaranteed to suffer a heart attack—or that having "safe" levels means you won't. Unfortunately, the cholesterol myth is so firmly embedded in our minds that sweating over cholesterol numbers has become a national obsession. Millions of people have been put on cholesterol-lowering drugs unnecessarily, while many more who could benefit from the medicines have not. The myth that cholesterol is always bad for you has led to related myths, like eating red meat or eggs is bad solely because they will increase your total cholesterol.

Let's sweep these myths aside once and for all. Cholesterol is *not* inherently bad, and an elevated level is not a sure sign of coronary heart disease—any more than low levels are a promise of heart health.

WHAT IS CHOLESTEROL?

Cholesterol is a natural, absolutely necessary substance manufactured by the body that is used to create bile acids, cell membranes, vitamin D, steroid hormones, testosterone, progesterone, and estrogen and to perform other vital tasks. It belongs to the lipid family of substances, which means it's a biochemical cousin of fat. Indeed, doctors use the term *dyslipidemia* to cover problems with cholesterol and blood fat as well as related items.

Cholesterol is a biological necessity, not a villain. Without ample amounts of the substance, you would die. Neither is modestly or even moderately elevated cholesterol a villain, for extra cholesterol floating through the bloodstream is not necessarily harmful to the arteries. In fact, in some cases the increase in cholesterol could be the body's way of trying to protect you from toxins or chronic infections. It's only when certain other things go wrong that cholesterol becomes problematic. Before looking at what these are, let's step back and learn a bit about cholesterol.

Most of the cholesterol inside you was manufactured by your body, with a smaller amount coming from your food. Cholesterol travels through your bloodstream to reach its various workstations. However, it's a fatty substance, while the blood is watery. Since fat and water don't mix, the body packages cholesterol, along with fats (triglycerides) and phospholipids, into different "containers" made of proteins for transport through the bloodstream. You can think of these as tiny submarines zipping around in your bloodstream, with different kinds of subs used for different kinds of cargo.

There are different versions of these containers, which are called lipoproteins, and they vary according to the ratio of protein, cholesterol, and fat they contain.

- Those with *more* protein and less cholesterol/fat are denser than the others, so they are called high-density lipoproteins, or HDL.
- Those with *less* protein and more cholesterol/fat are less dense, so they are known as low-density lipoproteins, or LDL.

- A third type, called very-low-density lipoprotein, or VLDL, carries even less protein and more cholesterol/fat.

According to standard thinking, LDL cholesterol is "bad" because it deposits cholesterol and fat in the arteries, while HDL is "good" because it acts like a garbage truck, snatching up cholesterol and fat from the arteries and carrying it away. Thus, you want to keep your LDL low and your HDL high. Your total cholesterol, which is a combination of the various types, should also be kept low.

When this theory was devised decades ago, it was the best way to explain what we knew about the relationship between cholesterol and heart disease. But it was very limited, for it rested on two major assumptions: first, that HDL, LDL, VLDL, and total cholesterol were far and away the major risk factors for heart disease and, second, that every single HDL particle was identical and that the same held true for LDL and VLDL. We've since learned that this is not true but have not revised the theory.

WHAT EVERYONE REALLY NEEDS TO KNOW ABOUT CHOLESTEROL

There is no single thing called HDL any more than there is just one item called LDL or VLDL. And the various cholesterol particles are not fixed and unchanging. Instead, there are different types of HDL, LDL, and VLDL, and they are constantly in flux, taking on different shapes and properties in response to their changing roles as well as to changing conditions in the body.

HDL comes in *at least* five distinct forms. The two most important of these are HDL-2 and HDL-3. They're both HDL, but HDL-2 is larger and more buoyant, while HDL-3 is smaller and denser.

This distinction is not just of interest to lab scientists peering through their electron microscopes, for HDL-2, especially the variety known as HDL-2B, offers more protection than HDL-3, so no matter how high or low your overall level of HDL, if you have ample amounts of HDL-2B, your risk of heart disease falls. On the other hand, if your levels of HDL-2 and HDL-2B levels are low, you are at risk of developing coronary heart disease, even if your total cholesterol and LDL cholesterol numbers are in the "safe" range. This means you could be put on a medicine because your overall HDL level is low, or not given medicine because it is high, even though your doctor may have absolutely no idea whether you have adequate amounts of the protective forms of HDL!

HDL size is largely inherited, but several things can increase the amount of the protective HDL-2 and HDL-2B in your blood, including exercising; losing weight; giving up smoking; restricting refined carbohydrates, trans fats, and saturated fats; and increasing your intake of niacin, omega-3 fatty acids, and pantethine.

LDL is also composed of different types that come in three different forms:

- *Lipoprotein(a)*—A "regular" LDL with a certain protein structure attached. The combination of the two increases the risk of developing clogged arteries and blood clots. The level of lipoprotein(a) is largely determined by genetics.
- *IDL (Intermediate-Density Lipoprotein)*—A VLDL that is depositing some of its cholesterol and fat in the arteries. Shedding the cholesterol and fat makes it more dense, so the VLDL "graduates" to the LDL category.
- *LDL-Real (LDL-R)*—All the remaining LDL.

These are all forms of LDL, but they behave differently in the body and need to be looked at individually when doctors are assessing the risk of heart disease. But they're usually not, for most lab tests simply report back a single LDL result that combines all three forms.

To make matters more complex, some LDL-R particles are large, others are small, and still others are somewhere in between. The large ones, which carry more cholesterol, are "fluffy" and more buoyant, while the small ones, which contain less cholesterol, are denser. The smaller ones are more dangerous, even though they contain less cholesterol, because they are better able to slip through the endothelium and burrow into artery walls. They are also more likely to be oxidized, which makes them even more dangerous. Once they're oxidized, glycated, or acetylated, they set in motion a series of events that acts as a biochemical magnet. They attract more inflammatory and other cells and particles to the toxic brew within the artery wall, raising the risk of a rupture, which can lead to a blood clot and a heart attack.

I remember two patients who had the exact same LDL level—100 mg/dL. But while Alan's LDL was composed mostly of large particles, Emily's LDL particles were mostly small, significantly increasing her risk of developing heart disease. But according to the standard LDL test, she and Alan were equally healthy. Emily clearly needed to begin treatment immediately but didn't because her doctor thought her LDL level was safe. Neither she nor her physician had any idea there was a problem inside her coronary arteries until she suffered a mild heart attack. Knowing that there are different forms and weights of LDL, it doesn't make sense to rely on a single number to determine whether someone is healthy. Yet we do.

Don't worry about memorizing all this. The point is that there is much more to HDL and LDL than your doctor saying your levels are "high" or "low." Physicians should be measuring the size and number of particles of the various types of HDL and LDL, but most routine cholesterol tests give only a single number representing the overall HDL or LDL level. The number of LDL particles is a key issue, for even if two people have the same LDL level, the person who has more LDL particles making up that number is at greater risk of developing coronary heart disease.

HOW CHOLESTEROL CONTRIBUTES TO CORONARY HEART DISEASE

The key point about cholesterol and heart disease is that certain forms of cholesterol—and *only* those forms—can slip past the endothelium in an area where a "scratch" has occurred, burrow into the artery wall, and make the toxic brew bubble even more dangerously. They do so by increasing the inflammation level and encouraging the oxidation that makes other particles more dangerous.

As for the rest of the cholesterol—the part floating through your bloodstream—it's not a threat to heart health as long as it stays in the bloodstream and does not build to wildly high numbers. We used to believe that when the total cholesterol number rose above a certain level, it somehow got "crammed" into the artery walls. But now we know that as long as there's no scratch and no bubbling cauldron inside an artery wall, you can tolerate quite a bit of cholesterol in your bloodstream— much more than most doctors realize.

When the "Good" HDL Goes Bad

One of the ways in which HDL can become harmful has to do with oxidation, which we talked about in chapter four.

Normally, HDL contains generous amounts of antioxidant substances and is an anti-inflammatory. But should inflammation levels rise too high, HDL can "flip" and become proinflammatory, filled with pro-oxidant molecules that interfere with HDL as it attempts to quell inflammation and oxidation and perform its other tasks. This, of course, increases the coronary heart disease risk.

New tests being developed will be able to detect this proinflammatory HDL and more accurately determine the risk of coronary heart disease.

HOW DO YOU KNOW WHETHER YOUR CHOLESTEROL IS IN THE DANGER ZONE?

Years ago, we looked only at total cholesterol, treating this single number as if it were a pronouncement from heaven saying either "You are at risk of having a heart attack" or "Don't worry, you're safe." As we learned more about cholesterol and how it functioned, we realized we had to look at the HDL, LDL, VLDL, and blood fat levels, along with the total cholesterol—the Big Five of lipids. Our knowledge has advanced considerably in the past decade, so it's time to go beyond the Big Five to look at dozens of cholesterol "fractions" and associated particles, including these:

- *Overall Number of LDL Particles*—Standard LDL tests measure only the LDL-C, or how much cholesterol is in a person's LDL. This is certainly an important number, but more significant is the number of LDL particles. To put it simply, the risk of suffering coronary heart disease increases as the particle number increases. Indeed, the LDL particle count is one of the best predictors of coronary heart disease. The levels should be less than 900 particles per mg/dL.

- *Sizes and Types of LDL "Bad" Cholesterol*—There are at least five types and sizes of LDL: the smallest size, type B, is the most dangerous, while the largest, type A, is the least harmful. The level of oxidized LDL is important, as is the number of LDL-B particles.[1]
- *VLDL or Triglycerides (Blood Fats)*—Excessive triglyceride levels increase the risk of clotting and atherosclerosis. Ideally, the triglyceride level should be below 75 mg/dL. If it is above 150 mg/dL, it should be investigated to see if the more dangerous aspects of VLDL are present, such as large VLDL particles and/or an increased number of VLDL particles and remnant VLDL particles.
- *HDL Cholesterol*—There are several types of HDL. The larger HDL-2B is most protective, while the smaller HDL-3 is least protective against coronary heart disease. The HDL-2B level should be above 40 mg/dL in men and 50 mg/dL in women. The ideal level is about 80 mg/dL.
- *Lipoprotein(a) (Lp(a))*—Lp(a) is a type of LDL that increases the risk of heart disease. Normal levels are usually less than 30 mg/dL.
- *Apolipoprotein B*—This carrier protein helps LDL deposit cholesterol in artery walls. The level should be less than 60 mg/dL and correlates with the LDL particle number.

In addition, your physician can learn more about your risk of coronary heart disease by testing your levels of the following substances:

- *Paraoxonase*—An enzyme that prevents the oxidation of HDL and the subsequent inflammation it can cause
- *Apolipoprotein C-II*—A protein that helps break apart VLDL and the fat particles called chylomicrons
- *Apolipoprotein A-I and A-II*—Protein complexes that carry HDL in the blood

- *Serum Free Fatty Acids*—Fat in the blood that takes the form of tiny, free-floating particles that increase the risk of coronary heart disease

These are key items physicians should be looking at when trying to determine if a patient's cholesterol, blood fat, and related substances are posing a danger—not just the potentially misleading total cholesterol, LDL, and HDL numbers.

NATURAL WAYS TO COMBAT THE DANGERS POSED BY HARMFUL FORMS OF CHOLESTEROL

There are many foods and supplements that can reduce total cholesterol or LDL cholesterol, and/or increase HDL cholesterol, including niacin, omega-3 fatty acids, pantethine, plant sterols, and the tocotrienols (forms of vitamin E). Exercise is also helpful in that regard, so simply following my Integrative Cardiovascular Disease Prevention Program will be very helpful for you.

Here are some of the elements of the program that deal with specific problems linked to cholesterol.

Cutting Back on Trans-Fatty Acids and Refined Carbohydrates

Fatty acids, the building blocks of fat, combine in different ways to produce different types of fat, just as amino acids join in various combinations to produce different proteins.

Almost all of the fats found in natural foods are made up of cis-fatty acids, which means the fatty acid is "kinked" and pliable. But when fat is manipulated to make processed and fast foods, some of these cis-fatty acids are converted into trans-fatty acids, which means they become "flat" and "straight."

This is good for food processors but bad for health, for trans-fatty acids are more likely to build up in the body and cause a number of problems.[2] They may:

- change the forms of cholesterol to more unfavorable types by inhibiting various enzymes
- lower levels of protective HDL (2 to 3 percent)
- increase apolipoprotein B (up to 8 percent)
- increase lipoprotein(a) (up to 4 percent)
- increase total cholesterol (up to 8 percent)
- increase LDL cholesterol (up to 9 percent)
- increase triglycerides and VLDL (up to 9 percent)
- increase the risk of developing a blood clot
- increase the risk of suffering from coronary heart disease and heart attack
- increase the risk of developing irregular heartbeat and suffering sudden death
- increase the risk of developing elevated blood pressure
- increase the likelihood of becoming obese

Eating foods containing trans-fatty acids leads to a buildup of these harmful substances in your fat tissue, leading to more inflammation and oxidative stress. As they continue to accumulate, a reserve of trans fats is built up and released for a long time, even after you stop consuming them.

Where We Get Trans-Fatty Acids

Trans-fatty acids are found in products containing hydrogenated fats, most notably margarine, shortening, and hydrogenated or partially hydrogenated oils. Thus, trans-fatty acids are found in doughnuts, cookies, cakes, potato chips, crackers, and other foods made with these kinds of fat. They are also found in deep-fried foods, French fries, and other foods fried in hydrogenated oils—often the case with fast food.

Avoiding Trans-Fatty Acids and Refined Carbohydrates

All packaged food products must list their trans fats content on the Nutrition Facts panel, so always check the label. If you see the words "hydrogenated" or "partially hydrogenated," you can be sure the food contains trans-fatty acids and should be avoided. Stay away from shortening, hydrogenated oils, margarine made with hydrogenated oil, and fried foods in general, especially those from fast food chains. If you like margarine, you can find several that are yogurt-based, "light," or contain omega-3 fatty acids and do not contain trans-fatty acids. Reduce all refined carbohydrates such as bread, white potatoes, pasta, rice, sweets, and sodas.

Drinking Green Tea

Green tea, which is made from the leaves of the *Camellia sinensis* plant, is a superior source of a group of naturally occurring flavonoids called catechins. The health-promoting effects of green tea's catechins have been widely studied over the past four decades, revealing that they have anticancer, antibacterial, and antiobesity effects. But perhaps most interesting is their wide-ranging protective effects against heart disease, which include the following:[3]

- reducing the oxidation of LDL
- decreasing secretion of apolipoprotein B, which means less is available to help LDL deposit cholesterol into artery walls
- lowering harmful LDL cholesterol while raising protective HDL cholesterol

Adding Green Tea to Your Diet

Green tea is mild, tasty, and refreshing, so it shouldn't be too hard to incorporate it into your diet. Have a cup first thing in the morning, and sip it throughout the day. Since it is quite low in caffeine, it probably won't make you jittery or sleepless. The goal is to get 500 milligrams of EGCG twice a day, which is easiest to achieve by taking supplements and drinking several cups of green tea throughout the day.

Consuming Omega-3 Fatty Acids

The omega-3 fatty acids found in cold-water fish and certain other foods first garnered attention when researchers noted that the Inuit rarely suffer from heart disease, despite the fact that they consume very large amounts of fat. But the fat they consume comes from fish and seals, rather than from beef or fried foods, and contains large amounts of omega-3 fatty acids. It soon became apparent that omega-3s protected the arteries and the heart.

Studies have shown that the omega-3 fatty acids can reduce the risk of coronary heart disease by, among other things,

- increasing levels of protective HDL-2
- increasing LDL particle size
- decreasing LDL particle number

In addition, they help reduce the inflammation that both creates and keeps the toxic brew bubbling inside the arterial wall, reverse endothelial dysfunction, and help the body create stronger "caps" to keep the toxic brew walled off inside the arterial wall so it can't come into contact with the blood.

Adding Omega-3 Fatty Acids to Your Diet

Omega-3 fatty acids are found primarily in cold-water fatty fish, such as salmon, mackerel, herring, and tuna. Be aware that fish raised on fish farms are lower in omega-3s than wild-caught fish due to the content of their diets. Other sources of omega-3s include fish oil, krill, and algae.

Precursors of omega-3s are flax, flaxseed, and flax oil, but eating these are less efficient ways of getting omega-3s into your system, as the body has to convert them. Not only is the conversion to DHA and EPA less than 5 percent, but these precursors may go into the inflammatory omega-6 pathway instead, increasing inflammation and coronary heart disease risk in some patients. Flax oil is not recommended.

The goal is a daily intake of 3 to 4 grams of EPA and DHA combined in a ratio of 3 parts EPA to 2 parts DHA. A 3-ounce serving of Pacific herring or Pacific oysters provides about 1.8 grams of EPA/DHA in the recommended ratio, while a 3-ounce serving of chinook salmon provides about 1.5 grams. Supplements of fish oil can make up the shortfall. It's also recommended that the 3 to 4 grams of EPA/DHA be balanced with 1.5 to 2 grams (about 50 percent of that total) gamma-linolenic acid (GLA) and 400 milligrams gamma-/delta-tocopherol vitamin E daily.

Additional Recommendations

Cutting back on trans-fatty acids and refined carbohydrates, drinking green tea, and consuming more omega-3 fatty acids will go a long way toward encouraging the manufacture of the helpful parts of cholesterol and discouraging the harmful ones. Adding in exercise will help more. For people who need even more, I recommend supplements such as the following:

1. Niacin: 100 milligrams per day to begin

A member of B family of vitamins that is also known as vitamin B_3, niacin has been used to promote heart health since the mid-1900s. Although it has been pushed aside by cholesterol-lowering medications, niacin's ability to lower cholesterol is widely recognized. The vitamin does the following:

- lowers small, dense LDL, shifts the harmful LDL-B pattern to the better LDL-A pattern, and reduces the LDL particle number
- reduces lipoprotein(a)
- lowers apolipoprotein B
- increases the helpful HDL-2B

Niacin should always be taken with food. Begin with 100 milligrams a day, slowly increasing the dose by 100 milligrams per week until a good response occurs. It is helpful to take a baby aspirin every day prior to the niacin, to help reduce flushing. Eating an apple or applesauce also helps reduce flushing. Do not drink alcohol at the same time you take niacin.

Niacin's potential side effects include flushing, itching, rash, liver dysfunction, high uric acid levels, and elevated blood sugar. Most of these are dose-related side effects, so beginning with a small dose and monitoring your reaction carefully as you increase it will help you catch any side effects early on and counter them by reducing the dose. Also remember that the "nonflush" niacin supplements sold over the counter do not work. They are composed of a different compound called IHN and, when compared with flush niacin (vitamin B_3) in clinical studies, are ineffective.

2. Tocotrienols: 100 milligrams daily of gamma-/delta-tocotrienols

Vitamin E is not a single substance. Instead, it is a group of eight substances with similar actions in the body. The eight substances are divided into two groups, called tocotrienols and tocopherols.

Studies have shown that the tocotrienols can improve the cholesterol situation by reducing harmful apolipoprotein B, lowering LDL and triglycerides, and increasing HDL. They also have antioxidant properties[4] that can help combat the oxidation that converts LDL into a more dangerous form.

I recommend a supplement containing 100 milligrams of gamma-/delta-tocotrienols. Take it with your evening meal, and make sure that twelve hours have passed since taking any other form of vitamin E.

3. Pantethine: 900 milligrams per day

A derivative of pantothenic acid (vitamin B_5), pantethine has numerous helpful properties, including[5]

- lowers apolipoprotein B up to 27.6 percent
- increases apolipoprotein A-I
- increases HDL
- lowers LDL and triglycerides

Pantethine also reduces the deposition of fats and the development of fatty streaks in the aorta and coronary arteries, reduces arterial wall thickening in the aorta and coronary arteries, and slows the oxidation of LDL into its more dangerous form.

Take 300 milligrams of pantethine three times a day or 450 milligrams twice a day. Peak effects usually occur after four months of supplementation, but it may take six to nine months to see them.

4. Polyphenols and Resveratrol: 250 milligrams per day

Polyphenols are naturally occurring compounds with powerful antioxidant properties found in green tea, apples, olive oil, walnuts, pomegranates, cocoa, and other foods of plant origin. One of the more famous polyphenols is resveratrol, which is found in the skin of grapes, purple grape juice, red wine, peanuts, and some berries. Research into polyphenols in general and resveratrol in particular has shown that they:

- reduce LDL oxidation
- increase the activity of a liver enzyme (PON-1) that helps prevent the oxidation of HDL
- reduce inflammation
- have antioxidant properties
- improve endothelial dysfunction

Only take resveratrol in the trans-resveratrol form, 250 milligrams per day, purchased from a highly reputable source such as Biotics Research. Do not take more than this, for clinical studies suggest that humans have the best response to this specific dose.

IT'S NOT JUST ONE NUMBER!

Between cutting back on trans-fatty acids, drinking green tea, consuming omega-3 fatty acids, and perhaps taking niacin, tocotrienols, pantethine, and resveratrol, you should be able to restore a healthy balance among the various types of cholesterol and related items.

The key point to remember is that the "cholesterol story" cannot be told simply by measuring total cholesterol, LDL, and HDL. *All* of the elements related to cholesterol must be measured to clearly identify the risk predictors—or to say with any certainty that one is in the "safe" zone.

Chapter Six

Maintaining Proper Blood Flow Through the Arteries

JUST AS CARS CAN damage the roads they ride on, blood can harm the arteries through which it flows. Blood moving through at just the right pressure and in exactly the right manner isn't a problem, but blood doesn't always flow in a perfect textbook way. Alterations in the speed or manner in which the blood flows through the coronary arteries raise the risk of heart disease, primarily by damaging the endothelium. The "scratches" this leaves in the artery walls are perfect places for the onset of inflammation and oxidative stress, plus the build-up of plaque, which can lead to atherosclerosis, blood clots, and blockages.

Prodded by physicians who are genuinely concerned about the very real link between high blood pressure (hypertension) and coronary heart disease, millions of Americans are taking beta-blockers, diuretics, calcium channel blockers, ACE inhibitors, and other medicines to reduce their blood pressure. For many patients, these medications are necessary and helpful, even lifesaving—but for others they are not. And some are at risk of potentially serious side effects. The diuretics, for example, can cause type 2 diabetes and high blood sugar, kidney insufficiency, increased uric acid levels and gout, and low potassium, while the beta-blockers can trigger fatigue, impotence, memory loss, insulin resistance, type 2 diabetes, low HDL cholesterol, and more. And due to genetic factors, many patients do not benefit much, if at all, from these medicines.

Ironically, many of the blood pressure medications, including certain diuretics and beta-blockers, can ratchet up other coronary heart disease risk factors. They may increase total cholesterol, LDL cholesterol, and triglyceride levels; lower HDL cholesterol; increase blood sugar levels; promote insulin resistance; and increase the risk of type 2 diabetes. Some diuretics can trigger kidney failure and lower levels of potassium, magnesium, and other nutrients. This negates their positive effects on reducing blood pressure and the risk of heart attack. Beta-blockers may only marginally reduce the risk of heart attack and stroke yet deplete the body of vital nutrients such as coenzyme Q10.

Medicines can be very helpful, but they're not always the best response to elevated blood pressure, and they're often given before the nature of the blood pressure problem and its effects on the endothelium have been explored. Before looking at ways to address these issues, let's take a look at what blood pressure is and how it causes "faulty arteries," or endothelial damage.

WHAT IS BLOOD PRESSURE?

You might think that all of the pressure within the cardiovascular system comes from the "push" generated by the beating of the heart, rather like the pressure in your house pipes being created by distant water pumps. That's not the case, for your arteries themselves contribute to the pressure. Unlike the pipes in your house, your blood vessels are active and dynamic.

The arteries in your heart and the rest of your body have tiny muscles built right into their walls. When the muscles in a given part of an artery contract, they squeeze the artery and narrow its diameter—just as a hose narrows when you step on it. When the muscles relax, the artery opens wide again. The arteries were designed this way to allow the nervous system to alter the flow of blood on command. Thus, if you suddenly find yourself facing an angry tiger, your nervous system causes arterial muscles to relax and contract in such a way as to slow the flow of blood to your stomach and other temporarily non-essential areas and shunt more to your large muscles, allowing you to either defend yourself or run away.

These arterial muscles contract and relax in response to what you're doing or thinking at any given moment, which means the arteries are continually opening wider or narrowing a bit. And with each muscular squeeze or relaxation, the blood pressure exerted in that area of the artery increases or decreases. This is called arterial compliance—the ability of the arteries to comply with, or cooperate with, your body's needs.

Back in medical school, I learned a simple formula: pressure equals force times resistance. As far as blood pressure is concerned, force is the amount of "oomph" created by the heart as it beats, while the resistance is the degree of push-back blood encounters as it passes through the arteries. If, for example, the arterial muscles are relaxed, allowing the arteries to open wide, and there is no plaque buildup or other obstructions in the arteries, there will be little or no resistance to the flow of blood, and blood pressure will be lower. But if the arterial muscles are contracting and narrowing the artery, and/or there are thick plaques on the arterial wall or other types of resistance, blood pressure will rise.

Interpreting the Numbers

Blood pressure readings are expressed as two numbers with a slash between them, as in 120/80, 100/70, 157/110, and so on. Two numbers are required because the blood pressure is not steady, like the pressure in your kitchen pipes when you turn on the water in the sink. Instead, it constantly increases and decreases as the heart beats and relaxes.

When the heart beats, the blood pressure goes up, and when it rests between beats, blood pressure drops. The pressure reading at the moment the heart is beating, called the systolic pressure, is the larger number, while the pressure reading at the moment the heart is relaxing, called the diastolic pressure, is the smaller number. The difference between the systolic and diastolic blood pressure is called the pulse pressure.

WHAT MAKES THE PRESSURE RISE?

Blood pressure is created by the force of the heart's pumping action and the resistance to blood flow offered by the arteries, which raises this question: What increases the heart's pumping action and/or the arterial resistance?

There's a long list of items that can increase the "push" or the resistance, including:

- caffeine—about 60 percent of the population has a genetic abnormality that slows the metabolism of caffeine in the liver, leading to an increased risk of elevated blood pressure
- low blood levels of vitamins C, D, and E
- elevated levels of iron in the blood
- low blood levels of magnesium
- low blood levels of coenzyme Q10—this substance spurs the production of adenosine triphosphate (ATP), which is

necessary for the heart's pumping action and blood flow in the coronary arteries
- low blood levels of lycopene
- smoking—inhalation, whether active or passive, of any kind of cigarette, pipe, or cigar smoke raises the blood pressure and harms the cardiovascular system in numerous ways
- high levels of stress—stress can flood the body with stress hormones, which increase the heart's pumping action
- proliferation/growth in vascular and heart muscle— unwanted growth in the arteries may make them thick, stiff, inelastic, and narrow, which increases blood pressure
- elevated levels of uric acid in the blood
- consumption of excessive amounts of trans-fatty acids
- obesity

These are certainly not the only things that can elevate blood pressure; there are also many medications, certain diseases, and other factors. But even this brief list gives you an idea of how easy it is to upset the delicate balance of "push" and resistance within the cardiovascular system, leading to changes in blood pressure.

HOW DOES RISING BLOOD PRESSURE HARM THE HEART?

Thanks to decades of exciting research, we now know that hypertension is a complex disease caused by a constellation of factors. In other words, it's not just a matter of consuming too much salt or suffering from too much stress. We now understand that hypertension, like coronary heart disease, begins in the arteries with increased oxidative stress, autoimmune dysfunction, and inflammation and that it is much more than a disease; it's a syndrome that incorporates and interacts with numerous disease states.

Elevated blood pressure is linked to problems in the arteries and kidneys, alterations in the way the body handles blood sugar and fats, changes in the structure and function of the heart, and much more. Rising pressure also increases the amount of inflammation and oxidative stress within the arteries, causes the endothelium to thicken, and increases autoimmune dysfunction of the arteries. And once hypertension begins, it contributes to the growth of some of these same harmful states, setting up a bidirectional negative feedback loop that can lead to disaster.

For example, endothelial dysfunction can interfere with the arteries' ability to contract and relax at the appropriate times, elevating the blood pressure. The blood pressure will rise, and the extra force exerted on the endothelium can further damage it and increase the endothelial dysfunction—which just makes the blood pressure go even higher.

In sum, elevated blood pressure increases damage to the endothelium, making it harder for the endothelium to perform all the tasks necessary to keep the cardiovascular system healthy and functioning.

HOW CAN YOU REALLY TELL IF YOUR BLOOD PRESSURE IS A PROBLEM?

Elevated blood pressure, or hypertension, is defined as elevated systolic pressure (more than 120 mm Hg), elevated diastolic blood pressure (more than 80 mm Hg), or both. Elevations of both systolic and diastolic blood pressure increase the risk for heart disease, but diastolic pressure is a better predictor of heart disease before the age of fifty-five, while systolic pressure is a better predictor of heart disease after the age of fifty-five.

Unfortunately, detecting elevated blood pressure or problems with blood flow within the arteries is not a simple matter of sliding the cuff onto your arm, pumping it up, releasing the cuff pressure slowly, and listening through a stethoscope to the sound of the blood as it moves through your arm. A single blood pressure reading taken at a doctor's office can be misleading, for it might be skewed by "white coat hypertension" and will certainly miss potentially dangerous changes in blood pressure that occur "silently" during the night. Blood pressure problems beyond the numbers include the following:

- *Widened Pulse Pressure*—The pulse pressure, which is difference between the two blood pressure numbers, is usually about 40. A higher pulse pressure is a sign of stiff arteries.
- *White Coat Hypertension*—These are elevations in blood pressure that occur when you go to the doctor's office but not when you're at home. This was previously thought to be due to nerves and considered harmless, but recent studies suggest that white coat or stress-induced hypertension may increase coronary heart disease and stroke risk.
- *Masked Hypertension*—This is the opposite of white coat hypertension. It is blood pressure that is normal in the physician's office but increased at home or when checked with twenty-four-hour blood pressure monitoring. This raises the risk of coronary heart disease.
- *Blood Pressure Dipping*—Those whose blood pressure dips (drops) about 10 percent at night have a lower risk of heart disease and stroke, while those whose pressure does not dip are at higher risk. Some patients dip too much, and this can also increase risk of coronary heart disease and stroke. Others have reverse dipping at night, which also increases risk.

- *Wide Fluctuations in Blood Pressure*—Extreme variations in blood pressure over a twenty-four-hour period increase the risk of heart attack and stroke.

- *Morning Surges in Blood Pressure*—Blood pressure typically increases early in the morning, even before you get out of bed, as your body prepares itself for the day. This is part of the circadian rhythm. A safe increase is less than 5 percent. More than a 20-percent increase suggests danger.

- *Hypertensive Response to Exercise*—The systolic blood pressure normally increases with exercise, but not much over 180 mm Hg. (The diastolic blood pressure falls or stays the same with exercise.) A systolic pressure that climbs too high or a diastolic pressure that increases at all indicates endothelial dysfunction, loss of arterial elasticity, and a tendency toward hypertension. It also could indicate extremely poor cardiovascular conditioning. This is detected with a cardiac stress test, as well as with the twenty-four-hour ambulatory blood pressure monitoring (if the patient exercises during that period). A safe result is a systolic pressure less than 180 mm Hg and either no change or about a 10-percent decrease in the diastolic blood pressure.

- *Stress-Induced Hypertension*

- *Changes in Blood Pressure Due to Diet, Weight Loss, Exercise, Nutrients, and Medications*

A single blood pressure reading taken in the doctor's office will miss a great number of important clues, which is why people who have or are at risk of having blood pressure variations should have a twenty-four-hour ambulatory blood pressure monitoring. The procedure is simple: A blood pressure cuff is attached to your arm at the doctor's office, a small monitor is hooked to a belt, and the two are connected by a wire.

(You sleep with the device in place.) You can detach the cuff yourself at the end of the twenty-four hours and return it and the monitor to your doctor's office, where the information held in the monitor is fed into a computer.

Other tests can detect additional problems, such as alterations in the way blood pulses through your arteries, enlargement of the heart chamber (left ventricle) that pumps blood through the body, increased arterial stiffness, and calcification of the coronary arteries. (See appendix VII for brief descriptions of some of these tests.)

NATURAL WAYS TO HELP RELIEVE THE PRESSURE

Once you've undergone the appropriate tests of your blood pressure and flow, you can take steps to correct any problems. If your problem is severe, you may need to start on medicines right away. If not, you can try natural and proven methods, such as the diet and exercise plans I'll describe in chapters to come, as well as herbs and nutrients such as the following:

- *Cocoa and Dark Chocolate*—A stream of studies has shown that cocoa and dark chocolate can aid heart health by reducing blood pressure and the functioning of the coronary arteries, among other actions.
- *Coenzyme Q10 (CoQ10)*—This is a natural substance produced by the body that assists in many reactions. It reduces blood pressure as well as oxidized LDL and serves as an antioxidant. CoQ10 levels typically begin to fall at about age thirty, and a great many people have moderately or significantly low levels.
- *Flavonoids*—This is a large group of compounds with antioxidant and other health-protective effects found in

vegetables, fruits, tea, coffee, wine, and fruit juice. In addition to other helpful actions, they reduce blood pressure. Resveratrol is the best known of the flavonoids.

- *Garlic*—This tasty food lowers blood pressure while combating inflammation and oxidation.
- *Green Tea*—This natural and tasty substance's ability to reduce blood pressure was confirmed by a study that tracked more than 1,500 people in China, who did not have high blood pressure, over the course of several years. Those who drank 0.5 to 2.5 cups of green or oolong tea per day were 46 percent less likely to develop high blood pressure, while in those who drank more than 2.5 cups per day, the figure rose to 65 percent.
- *Hawthorn*—An herb used to treat various heart and cardiovascular ailments, hawthorn has been shown to reduce blood pressure, combat inflammation and oxidation, and reduce the risk of coronary heart disease.
- *Lutein*—A member of the carotenoid family and therefore related to vitamin A and beta-carotene, lutein lowers blood pressure and combats the oxidation of LDL. It's found in egg yolks; dark-green leafy vegetables; and tomatoes, carrots, corn, and other fruits and vegetables that contain red, orange, or yellow pigments. It is not manufactured by the body.
- *Lycopene*—A pigment that imparts a red color to watermelon, tomatoes, and other fruits and vegetables, lycopene is a member of the carotenoid family. In addition to lowering blood pressure, lycopene is an antioxidant and improves endothelial dysfunction.
- *Melatonin*—A hormone produced in the brain, melatonin lowers blood pressure along with oxidative stress and inflammation and improves endothelial dysfunction. In addition to being manufactured by the body, melatonin is found in vegetables, fruits, grains, and herbs.

- *Omega-3 Fatty Acids*—Studies have shown that these fatty acids can reduce elevated blood pressure.
- *Potassium*—This mineral helps counteract the tendency of salt to raise blood pressure in salt-sensitive people.
- *Resveratrol*—This substance, found in grapes, purple grape juice, red wine, peanuts, and some berries lowers blood pressure, combats endothelial dysfunction, and inhibits blood clots.
- *Sesamin*—Found in sesame, sesamin can help reduce elevated blood pressure. A 2006 paper published in the *Journal of Medicinal Food* reported on a study involving forty adults with mild to moderately elevated blood pressure and diabetes.[1] For forty-five days, the participants used sesame oil for all their cooking needs, and for another forty-five days they used palm or other oils. While they were cooking with sesame oil, their blood pressure and blood glucose levels dropped.
- *Vitamin C*—An antioxidant found in fresh fruits and vegetables, this vitamin reduces blood pressure and improves endothelial dysfunction and the ability of the arteries to stretch and contract on demand.
- *Vitamin D*—Although best known for strengthening the bones, this vitamin also helps regulate blood pressure.
- *Wakame Seaweed*—A thin, deep-green seaweed used for making miso soup and salad, wakame has been shown to reduce elevated blood pressure in human and animal studies.
- *Whey Protein*—Found in the liquid that remains after milk has been curdled and strained, whey protein contains peptides the serve as precursors to glutathione. It also lowers blood pressure.

RECOMMENDATIONS

If tests show you have hypertension or any problems with blood pressure or flow, I recommend you begin on this regimen immediately. Have your blood pressure and/or flow checked regularly to monitor your progress and adjust your program (and possibly medications) accordingly.

Daily Regimen

1. A Heart-Healthy Diet

My Integrative Cardiovascular Disease Prevention Program Diet is a modified version of the DASH II diet, which has been proven to help keep blood pressure under control. On this diet, you'll be consuming helpful nutrients, such as magnesium, potassium, vitamin B_6, vitamin C, vitamin D, fiber, and omega-3 fatty acids. You'll also be eating far fewer of the transfatty acids that encourage blood pressure to rise. (See chapter nine for a complete discussion of diet.)

2. Regular Exercise

Numerous studies have shown that regular exercise helps control elevated blood pressure. One of the ways it does so is by inducing weight loss, which in and of itself can tamp down blood pressure. (See chapter ten for a complete discussion of exercise for heart disease prevention, including my ABCT Exercise Program.)

3. Use of Supplements

I listed several key supplements above, and there are many more. Beginning with five or ten supplements at once can be overwhelming, so you might want to start with just a few, have your blood pressure checked regularly, and adjust as necessary. A simple way to start is with these three:

- cocoa—30 grams dark chocolate per day
- CoQ10—100 milligrams twice a day
- vitamin C—500 milligrams twice a day

4. Reduced Sodium Intake: maximum 1,500 milligrams per day

Although not everyone is sodium sensitive, it's a good idea to limit your daily intake to 1,500 milligrams a day. You'll have to get in the habit of reading the nutrition labels on all the foods you eat and liquids you drink to know how much you're consuming. Beware of fast foods, for they tend to have more sodium than you would suspect. A McDonald's hamburger, for example, has 520 milligrams of sodium, while a Double Quarter Pounder with Cheese has 1,380![2]

FOCUS ON THE BIGGER PICTURE

I began this book by critiquing the myth that coronary heart disease could be banished if we simply conquered the Big Five risk factors—one of which is elevated blood pressure. I stand by that statement, for focusing on the Big Five is misleading at best and dangerous at worst. That does not mean, however, that elevated blood pressure should be ignored or that disturbances in blood flow should be discounted. Blood pressure issues are more complicated than simply measuring your blood pressure in the doctor's office. It requires a twenty-four-hour blood pressure monitoring to identify some of the "hidden" issues within the blood pressure diagnosis, as well as other tests, including those that check the status of the arteries and endothelium, to determine your coronary heart disease risk and the type of treatment you need.

The important point to remember is that elevated blood pressure and disturbances in blood flow are both a cause and a result of endothelial dysfunction and should be viewed and treated within that context, rather than as isolated problems that can be identified with a single blood pressure reading.

Chapter Seven

Preventing Blood Sugar and Insulin from Harming the Heart

THE HUMAN BODY cannot survive without access to fuel in the form of sugar (glucose), and that sugar must be readily accessible. To ensure that cells can always and easily fuel up, the body wants to make sure there's plenty of sugar floating through the bloodstream at all times. This wouldn't be a problem if you ate continuously throughout the day and night, grazing on foods that provided just as much sugar as your body needed at the moment. You don't do this, of course. Instead, you eat three large meals and several liquid or solid snacks a day, which means you have plenty of sugar fuel in your body after you've eaten, but lesser amounts between meals and even less during the hours between your last meal of the day and the next morning's breakfast.

To make sure you always have exactly as much as you need, your body carefully regulates the level of sugar in the blood, storing the excess from meals in designated cells throughout the body. Unfortunately, it's not a simple matter of saying that X percent of the sugar from this meal goes into the blood while Y percent goes to storage—like putting 10 percent of your newly purchased groceries on the kitchen counter for meal preparation and the rest in the refrigerator. Instead, there's a complex system involving instructing cells to open their "doors" to the sugar—the conversion of sugar from one form to another as it goes from your food to your bloodstream to your storage cells and back to your bloodstream—and numerous helper substances to make sure the system works properly.

With complexity comes the increased possibility for errors and trouble to occur, and tens of millions of Americans are in blood sugar trouble. We typically call this trouble diabetes, and that's what physicians tend to focus on when thinking of coronary heart disease. But we need to go beyond thinking in terms of a single disease and begin to consider all the heart-related problems that blood sugar can cause or contribute to, including creating the toxic brew inside an artery wall, increasing the level of blood fats, and causing insulin resistance, which can trigger a long list of serious events.

WHAT'S THE LINK BETWEEN EXCESS BLOOD SUGAR AND CORONARY HEART DISEASE?

You might think that sugar is not dangerous; after all, it's simply fuel waiting to be used. But so is the gasoline that fuels our cars, and we take great pains to make sure that it is carefully stored, transferred to gas tanks in just the right way, and then handled precisely as it's burned for energy in the engine. We don't just open the hood and pour a few gallons onto the engine!

Trouble may begin as soon as you eat, for there is an inverse relationship between excess sugar from food (sucrose), HDL cholesterol, and triglycerides; that is, when sugar consumption rises, HDL decreases and triglycerides increase.

Problems continue if your body has difficulty stuffing blood sugar into storage cells. This is not an automatic process, a simple matter of pulling the plug on the bottom side of the arteries and letting the extra blood sugar drop into the storage cells. Instead, it's a carefully regulated process spearheaded by insulin, a hormone charged with the task of pushing the excess sugar into storage.

Some people don't make nearly enough insulin, or none at all, so they can't prevent sugar from rising to dangerously high levels in their blood. We call this problem type 1 diabetes, and it's treated with insulin injections that replace what the body cannot manufacture. For many more people, the problem isn't a lack of insulin, it's that their insulin doesn't do its job well. They have a problem known as insulin resistance, which means the storage cells resist the efforts of insulin to fill them with sugar. The body tries to overcome this problem by pumping out more and more insulin. It often succeeds in eventually cramming the excess sugar into storage. Unfortunately, the sugar-stuffing battle leaves its mark on the arteries, just as any earthly battlefield is damaged as two opposing armies pass over it. The combination of excess sugar floating through the arteries and the sugar-stuffing battle encourages inflammation, oxidative stress, autoimmune dysfunction of the arteries, and endothelial dysfunction—among other problems. This means elevated blood sugar is a risk factor for coronary heart disease.

The Key Point

You don't have to have full-blown diabetes for your arteries to be suffering. The damage starts sooner than that, with the development of insulin resistance and "prediabetes." Waiting to be diagnosed with diabetes and then treating it with medications solely designed to get blood sugar numbers back in line means doing too little, too late.

HOW DO YOU KNOW IF YOU HAVE A BLOOD SUGAR PROBLEM?

Ideally, you could take a simple, one-time-only blood test to get a definitive answer. Unfortunately, it's not just a matter of a good or bad blood sugar level at the moment you're in your doctor's office, for there are several factors to consider, including your blood sugar level immediately after eating and when fasting, as well as the effectiveness of your insulin. That's why your blood sugar should be tested both before and after you eat.

- *Before You Eat*—A fasting blood glucose test allows the doctor to determine how well your body handles the release of sugar from storage when no new sugar is coming in from food. Fasting blood sugar levels higher than 80 mg/dL should be considered abnormal.
- *After You Eat*—This is measured with a two-hour glucose tolerance test, which involves consuming a beverage containing a specific amount of sugar and tracking the change in your blood sugar over a set period of time. Results over 110 mg/dL are a cause for concern.

Unfortunately, you can be lulled into complacency by the way glucose levels are reported on laboratory reports. For example, most labs indicate that a fasting blood sugar up to 99 mg/dL is normal, so you probably won't worry much if your result is 100, just one point beyond the cutoff. However, starting at a fasting level of 80 mg/dL, each 1 mg/dL increase in glucose raises the risk of coronary heart disease by 1 percent, so a rise in fasting blood sugar from 80 to 100 means the risk of coronary heart disease increased by 20 percent! Your insulin level should be monitored in addition to your blood sugar level, for an elevated insulin level is a predictor of coronary heart disease, *even if the blood sugar level is normal.* If you have insulin resistance, your insulin level will rise dramatically as your body attempts to keep your blood sugar normal. Unfortunately, the presence of insulin resistance can alter the behavior of your heart, muscles, fat, kidneys, and other organs, triggering an increase in blood pressure, sodium, and water retention; dysfunction of the heart muscle; inflammation; dyslipidemia; coronary heart disease; and more.

Finally, it's worthwhile to check for elevations in your hemoglobin A1c (HbA1c), which shows how much blood glucose has been adhering to the oxygen-carrying hemoglobin molecules in your red blood cells over the long term. It reflects both your fasting and postmeal glucose levels. This test offers a look at the body's ability to control blood glucose over a period of about three months. Ideally, the result should be less than 5.5 percent.

A FEW WORDS ABOUT METABOLIC SYNDROME

The insulin resistance that characterizes type 2 diabetes—which millions of Americans have—is not an isolated problem that triggers a single disease. Instead, it is key factor in a constellation of problems that have been named metabolic syndrome (formerly known as syndrome X). Metabolic syndrome is a group of risk factors, including insulin resistance, excess weight around the midsection of the body (an apple-shaped body), and sedentary lifestyle, that dramatically increases the risk of developing type 2 diabetes, stroke, and coronary heart disease. To be diagnosed with metabolic syndrome, you must have at least three of the following five indicators:

1. abdominal obesity—storing excess fat around the midsection of the body, as opposed to the hips or other parts of the body
2. elevated blood fats (triglycerides)
3. low HDL cholesterol
4. elevated blood pressure
5. elevated fasting blood sugar

If you have insulin resistance or diabetes, ask your physician to look into the possibility that you have metabolic syndrome. If you have it, get treatment. And if you don't have it, do everything you can to ward it off.

WHAT INCREASES BLOOD SUGAR?

A number of things can push blood sugar up:

- *Excessive Intake of Refined Carbohydrates*—In addition to increasing blood sugar, consuming too many refined carbohydrates increases inflammation, oxidative stress, diabetes, and the risk of heart attack.
- *Anything More Than a Slight Intake of High-Fructose Corn Syrup (HFCS)*—This ubiquitous sweetener increases blood sugar and blood fats, induces inflammation and oxidative stress, and raises the risk diabetes mellitus, obesity, and heart disease.
- *Low Levels of Vitamin D*—A deficiency of this vitamin can lead to an increase in blood sugar, along with an elevated risk of insulin resistance, diabetes, and obesity.
- *Low Levels of Chromium and Other Micronutrients and Electrolytes*—Lack of the mineral chromium impairs insulin secretion and raises blood glucose. Low levels of potassium, magnesium, biotin, and other B vitamins can also increase glucose.

- *Elevated Serum Free Fatty Acids*—The number of these tiny, free-floating fat particles is especially elevated in those with insulin resistance, high blood glucose, and diabetes mellitus.
- *Numerous Medications*—Some medications, including certain diuretics and beta-blockers used for treating elevated blood pressure and certain heart problems, promote insulin resistance and increase the risk of type 2 diabetes.
- *Obesity*—Being significantly overweight may trigger insulin resistance, which, in turn, leads to problems controlling blood sugar.
- *Insulin Resistance*—This disease state elevates blood sugar and increases the risk of type 2 diabetes. It also drives endothelial dysfunction by inducing inflammation and increasing blood fat levels.
- *Low Skeletal Muscle Mass (Lean Body Mass)*—This hampers the ability of insulin to act, thereby increasing insulin resistance.
- *Low Testosterone Levels in Men*—This leads to decreased lean body muscle mass and increased body fat and insulin resistance.
- *Lack of Exercise and Sedentary Lifestyle*

NATURAL WAYS TO LOWER ELEVATED BLOOD SUGAR AND ADDRESS RELATED PROBLEMS

It's very important that your body's ability to control blood sugar and insulin be tested and, if either is less than optimal, that you take steps to correct the problem. If you have high blood sugar or diabetes, you might be tempted to rely solely on prescribed insulin. I know people who eat all the sugary and fatty foods they want, simply taking more insulin when they know they're "being bad."

Unfortunately, this approach won't quash all the damage being done to your arteries, and while medications can be helpful, every single one of them carries the risk of side effects. That's why, unless you've reached a critical point, it's often best to begin with natural methods, such as these food components and supplements, for treating elevated blood sugar and insulin resistance:

- *Chromium*—This mineral helps the body secrete the insulin necessary to control blood sugar.
- *Green Tea (EGCG Extract)*—This is tea made from the leaf of the *Camellia sinensis* bush. The active ingredients in green tea, called catechins, lower blood sugar levels and also improve endothelial dysfunction. EGCG is one of the key catechins.
- *Pycnogenol*—Made from the French maritime pine tree, this supplement lowers blood sugar and may also help slow endothelial damage.
- *Sesamin*—Found in sesame, sesamin helps reduce blood sugar. In 2006, an article published in the *Journal of Medicinal Food* reported on a study in which forty adults with mildly to moderately elevated blood pressure and diabetes were asked to cook with either sesame oil or other oils for forty-five days.[1] At the end of the study period, the researchers found that while the study participants were using sesame oil, their blood sugar (and blood pressure) levels dropped.
- *Soluble Fiber*—Found in greater amounts in whole grains, root vegetables, beans, and other foods, soluble fiber reduces blood glucose and insulin levels.
- *R-Lipoic Acid*—This is a form of the natural substance alpha-lipoic acid, which is produced in the human body and found in some food. Used as a supplement, r-lipoic acid improves insulin sensitivity and lowers glucose levels.

- *Cinnamon*—This popular spice lowers blood sugar levels in people with diabetes.
- *Biotin and B Vitamins*—A member of the B family of vitamins found in yeast, whole wheat bread, eggs, and other foods, biotin works with other B vitamins to regulate blood sugar levels.
- *Fenugreek*—An herb used in traditional Chinese medicine and ayurvedic medicine and found in curry, fenugreek contains the natural fiber galactomannan, which appears to interfere with the absorption of sugar from food.
- *Bitter Melon*—A tropical fruit, bitter melon helps the body move blood sugar into storage cells.
- *Potassium and Magnesium*—The mineral potassium helps the body convert blood sugar into glycogen, the form muscles can utilize. Magnesium, which participates in more than three hundred reactions in the body, helps control blood sugar levels and blood pressure. Low levels of magnesium, often found in those with type 2 diabetes, may make insulin resistance worse. It's best to get these minerals from foods, where they are in the presence of other nutrients in healthful ratios. Good sources of potassium include dried figs, avocado, papaya, dates, and bananas. Good sources of magnesium include avocado, tofu, almonds, filberts, and spinach.

RECOMMENDATIONS

If you already have diabetes or metabolic syndrome, you should be under a physician's care and following a strict, low-refined-carbohydrate diet; exercising; losing body fat; and possibly taking medications. In addition, begin on this daily regimen to help your body regain control. As your blood sugar and insulin levels return to normal, you can begin weaning yourself off medication with your doctor's help.

Daily Regimen

1. A Heart-Healthy Diet

The Integrative Cardiovascular Disease Prevention Program Diet I recommend to my patients eliminates much of the fast food, refined carbohydrates, and high-fructose corn syrup that contribute to elevated blood sugar. It also helps overcome insulin resistance by helping you slim down to a healthier weight. (See chapter nine for a complete discussion of the diet.)

2. Regular Exercise

Exercise lowers blood sugar, for it burns up the muscles' stores of sugar and forces them to take sugar out of the blood. When you've finished exercising, your liver takes even more sugar from the blood and makes it available as a ready reserve for the muscles. My ABCT Exercise Program will cause you to burn sugar already in your body and, by helping you shed excess pounds, will combat insulin resistance and help reverse or ward off metabolic syndrome. (See chapter eleven for a complete discussion of my ABCT Exercise Program.)

3. Chromium: 200 to 800 micrograms per day

Studies of people with diabetes have shown that taking this mineral in supplement form can reduce fasting blood sugar levels, after-meal blood sugar levels, and fasting insulin levels. The authors of a paper published in 2004 summed up their review of the literature by noting, "Growing evidence suggests that chromium supplementation, particularly at higher doses and in the form of [chromium picolinate], may improve insulin sensitivity and glucose metabolism in patients with glucose intolerance and type 1, type 2, gestational, and steroid induced diabetes."[2]

4. EGCG Extract: 500 milligrams twice per day

Epigallocatechin gallate (EGCG) is one of the health-enhancing catechins found in green tea. Human and animal studies indicate that EGCG can help lower blood sugar and improve the body's ability to properly handle blood sugar. In a study involving 17,413 middle-age people, green tea was found to reduce the risk of developing type 2 diabetes.[3] Dosage was important, with those drinking six cups of green tea or more per day being 33 percent less likely to develop diabetes than those consuming one cup per week or less. And in laboratory conditions testing EGCG specifically, this catechin slowed DNA fragmentation and other forms of cellular damage triggered by very high levels of glucose.[4]

5. Biotin: 10 to 15 milligrams per day

We've long known from animal studies that biotin plays a key role in the utilization of blood sugar, and human studies have shown biotin levels are lower in those with type 2 diabetes than in healthy people. The vitamin also helps control the elevation of blood fats seen with diabetes and, in animal studies, encourages the release of insulin.

THE DISEASE IS IN THE DETAILS

By the time diabetes has been diagnosed, there's a good chance that you've already suffered endothelial damage. And you'll probably continue to do so if all you do is take medications to get your blood sugar levels into the acceptable range.

Out-of-control blood sugar and insulin begin nibbling into cardiovascular health before they blossom into full-fledged disease—and when they do, they can combine with other factors to produce the even more threatening metabolic syndrome.

Don't wait to get tested, and don't wait to begin eating properly, exercising, and doing everything else you can to keep your blood sugar in the healthy zone and your arteries sound.

Chapter Eight

A Potpourri of Other Risk Factors

IN THE PREVIOUS CHAPTERS, we looked at key Fast Track to Heart Disease Pathways, how they contribute to cardiovascular disease, and what can be done to prevent or reverse the damage. In this chapter, I'll briefly review a host of other items, states, and diseases that can damage the arteries and set the stage for coronary heart disease.

There are literally hundreds of substances, states, conditions, and diseases that can harm the endothelium, including inflammation, oxidation, and disturbances in cholesterol, blood fat, blood pressure, and blood sugar, which we've already talked about. Sometimes the connection is obvious, while other times it is not. Obesity is a fast track for many reasons, including the fact that it can trigger significant "hidden" inflammation.

It's important to remember that many of the individual items are often just variations—minor changes in the body that aren't terribly harmful in and of themselves. It's only when they combine with your unique biochemistry, diet, and lifestyle that they become problematic. But if allowed to fester and grow, they invariably lead to arterial inflammation, oxidation, and problems with autoimmunity, and then you're faced with toxic brews within your arterial walls, alterations to blood pressure and flow, and other serious problems.

Before moving on, I'd like to spend a few moments looking at vascular autoimmunity, or problems with the behavior of the immune system in the arteries. The immune system is the body's built-in defender that attacks germs, viruses, cancer cells, and other dangers that make their way into or arise within the body. When it senses a danger, the immune system creates an antibody, T cell, or other substance that attacks the thing that is not a part of the healthy body.

With autoimmunity, the helpful process goes haywire. For example, the immune system may detect the presence of modified LDL, oxidized HDL, a heavy metal, or bacteria from periodontal disease; correctly identify it as a potential danger; then manufacture antibodies, cytokines, inflammatory substances, and oxidative molecules to destroy it. This is good, but the process is not perfect. Sometimes, the result is an "antigen-antibody complex," which arises when the defender latches onto the dangerous substance and refuses to let go. This renders the foreign substance helpless, but then something has to be done with the intertwined duo. The body may deposit it in the arteries to get rid of it, but there it can cause inflammation, oxidative stress, and arterial damage. As a result, the body is inadvertently harming the blood vessels.

Virtually all of the risk factors that cause inflammation and oxidative stress also produce autoimmune dysfunction of the arteries. This means if you have inflammation or oxidative stress in your arteries, there's a good chance you also have vascular autoimmunity. What causes inflammation and oxidative stress also causes vascular autoimmunity, and the things you do to reduce inflammation and oxidative stress also help calm the errant immune system.

Now let's take a look at several dozen other variations that can lead to coronary heart disease.

GENETIC VARIATIONS PATHWAYS

Certain inherited traits can increase the risk of coronary heart disease. There may be nothing that can be done about them, but it's helpful to know if you have these risk-increasing genetic variations. Then you can do everything possible to counteract the risk they pose by tamping down your other variations. These genetic variations include the following:

- *Family History of Premature Cardiovascular Disease*—If your father had a heart attack before the age of sixty or your mother had one before the age of fifty-five, you are at increased risk.
- *Male-Pattern Baldness*—There is an interesting association between male-pattern baldness and coronary heart disease, but we do not yet understand why they are linked, and one does not seem to cause the other.
- *Diagonal Earlobe Crease and Hairy Earlobes*—This is another interesting association, but not necessarily cause and effect. The mechanism is not known.
- *Short Stature*—In men less than about 5 feet 5 inches in height and women less than 5 feet tall, the risk for coronary heart disease is increased by about 50 percent.
- *Being Too Tall*—Men over 6 feet tall and women standing more than 5 feet 8 inches tall have an increased risk of coronary heart disease.
- *Single Nucleotide Polymorphisms (SNPs)*—More than seven hundred of these genetic variants, which can increase the risk of coronary heart disease, have been identified. They can harm heart health in a number of ways,

including interfering with the metabolism of cholesterol and HDL. (See chapter one for more on SNPs.)

NUTRITION AND RELATED VARIATIONS PATHWAYS

We've talked about nutrition in the previous chapters and will talk more about it in chapter nine. Here's a list to help you keep the nutrition variations in mind and give you an idea of how many factors are involved:

- *Caffeine Use*—About 60 percent of the population is at increased risk for atherosclerosis, heart attack, and other problems due to consumption of caffeine from any source. This is because of a genetic abnormality that slows the metabolism of caffeine in the liver, leading to an increased risk of coronary heart disease, heart attack, and high blood pressure.
- *Reduced Intake of Fruits and Vegetables*—The optimal daily intake is six servings of vegetables and four servings of fruit. Anything less than this may result in low levels of antioxidants in the blood.
- *Reduced Intake of Omega-3 Fatty Acids*—These are helpful fats the body needs to build good health. Found in cold-water fish, other foods, and nutritional supplements, the omega-3s help reduce inflammation and atherosclerosis, increase HDL and HDL-2B particles, reduce LDL particles, keep the heart beating regularly, and stabilize dangerous plaque. Thanks to these and other properties, omega-3s reduce the risk of coronary heart disease.
- *Reduced Intake of Polyunsaturated Fatty Acids (PUFAs) and Monounsaturated Fatty Acids (MUFAs)*—These include fats that contribute to heart and overall health.

- *Increased Intake of Trans-Fatty Acids*—Trans-fatty acids are fatty acids with an unusual molecular structure. Rarely found in nature, in the human diet they come almost entirely from processed foods in which a "bend" in the structure was deliberately straightened to change the fat's cooking, processing, or storage characteristics. That's good for food manufacturers but bad for us, for the altered fatty acids are very harmful to human health.

- *Increased Intake of Omega-6 Fatty Acids*—A type of fatty acid found in corn oil, sunflower seed oil, safflower oil, pumpkin seeds, baked goods, and other foods, the omega-6 fatty acids are natural substances that perform necessary duties in the body, such as serving as precursors for prostaglandins. Unfortunately, they can be harmful in the large quantities found in the typical American diet, being linked to inflammation, arthritis, obesity, breast cancer, and other ailments.

- *Low Blood Levels of Vitamin C*—An antioxidant, vitamin C helps to recycle other antioxidants, lowers blood pressure, protects the arteries, reduces arterial stiffness, and much more.

- *Low Blood Levels of Vitamin E*—Low antioxidant levels and the inability to protect cell membranes leads to oxidative stress and increases in blood pressure. As an antioxidant, vitamin E helps protect against these problems. Humans use the gamma-/delta-tocopherol form of vitamin E, which is the type found in our food, for metabolism. Vitamin E supplementation should be primarily of the gamma-/delta-tocopherol form.

- *Low Blood Levels of Vitamin K*—Vitamin K comes in multiple forms, and both vitamins K_1 and K_2 are important, especially the form known as vitamin K_2 MK7. This form of the vitamin protects the heart by serving as a cofactor for an enzyme that produces a protein that reduces arterial plaque formation and calcification—and may even reverse plaque formation and calcification in the coronary arteries.

- *Low Blood Levels of Chromium*—Chromium helps improve insulin resistance and glucose levels.
- *Low Blood Levels of Copper*—Small amounts of copper are needed for proper cell function and to reduce oxidative stress. Too much copper, however, can be dangerous, especially for men.
- *Low Blood Levels of Magnesium*—Magnesium lowers blood pressure, improves insulin resistance and glucose levels, reduces heart arrhythmias, improves endothelial dysfunction, decreases inflammation and oxidative stress, and lowers the risk of coronary heart disease.
- *Low Blood Levels of Lycopene*—Lycopene, a potent antiox idant and anti-inflammatory, lowers blood pressure while reducing coronary heart disease.
- *Low Blood Levels of Coenzyme Q10*—A potent antioxidant, CoQ10 reduces oxidative stress, inflammation, blood pressure, insulin resistance, glucose levels, and oxidation of LDL. It also improves ATP production for cellular energy, the heart's pumping action, and blood flow in the coronary arteries. All told, it reduces the risk of coronary heart disease and heart attack, and it improves congestive heart failure. CoQ10 is found in meat, some oils, fish, nuts, beans, chicken, eggs, and vegetables, but only in small amounts, so supplements are needed.
- *Elevated Blood Levels of Iron and Ferritin*—In men, elevated levels of iron can raise the risk of heart attack by increasing the oxidative stress and inflammation that cause endothelial dysfunction.

The levels of most of these substances can be measured in the blood, although they may vary from day to day, depending on what was eaten over the previous twenty-four hours. In addition, nutrient levels in the blood don't always accurately reflect the amounts that have made their way into the cells, and the "normal" levels reported on lab results may be inadequate for some people. For these reasons, standard blood tests may not give the most accurate view of nutrient levels.

A more scientifically accurate and medically useful approach is to determine if the cells have the nutrients they need for optimal functioning. I check this using the micronutrient test,[1] which measures twenty-eight micronutrients, including vitamins A, C, D, E, K; all the B vitamins (B_1, B_2, B_3, B_6, B_{12}, folate, pantothenate, and biotin); choline; carnitine; inositol; oleic acid; calcium; zinc; copper; magnesium; chromium; glutathione; cysteine; coenzyme Q10; selenium; lipoic acid; glucose and fructose sensitivity; amino acids such as asparagine, glutamine, and serine; and total antioxidant defense. This test of nutrient function within the cells is a better means of determining which nutrients are lacking and how they should be restored to optimal levels.

LIFESTYLE AND CULTURAL VARIATIONS PATHWAYS

A significant portion of the coronary heart disease risk is related to our modern lifestyle, much of which we can control. These controllable lifestyle predictors include the following:

- *Physical Inactivity/Lack of Exercise*—Lack of exercise encourages obesity, hypertension, elevated cholesterol, glucose, inflammation, and oxidative stress, which raise the risk of coronary heart disease.
- *Low Lean Muscle Mass and Decreased Muscle Strength in Men*[2]
- *Smoking*—Inhalation, whether active or passive, of any kind of cigarette, pipe, or cigar smoke increases the

tendency of the blood to clot, raises blood pressure, introduces free radicals, and harms the cardiovascular system in countless other ways.

- *Excessive Intake of Alcohol*—Excessive ingestion of alcohol increases blood pressure, blood fats, calorie intake, obesity, inflammation, and the risk for coronary heart disease and stroke. More than two drinks per day for men (20 grams of alcohol) and one for women (10 grams of alcohol) is excessive.
- *Chronic Lack of Sleep*—Sleeping less than six hours per night increases the risk of coronary heart disease and related problems. Eight hours per night appears to be the ideal amount of sleep. Ten hours is too much, as it increases the risk of stroke.[3]
- *Sleep Apnea*—This is a disorder in which breathing pauses during sleep, or the breathing rate becomes abnormally low. Sleep apnea increases the risk for obesity, diabetes, hypertension, coronary heart disease, irregular heartbeat, and stroke.

PSYCHOLOGICAL VARIATIONS PATHWAYS

The human mind and body are not separate and distinct entities but rather different aspects of a single unit. What happens to one always influences the other. Mind-related conditions that can harm the coronary arteries and heart health include the following:

- *High Levels of Stress*—Stress can cause anxiety, depression, insomnia, changes in mood and physiology (such as increased heart rate and blood pressure), and changes in hormones (such as increased cortisol and adrenalin).
- *Chronic Anxiety*
- *Chronic Depression*

- *Hostility*
- *Type A Personality (Aggressive Subtype)*—This is a behavioral pattern characterized by high levels of impatience, aggressiveness, tension, a need to control others, and difficulty relaxing. It elevates the levels of hormones such as cortisol and adrenalin, as well as cytokines and inflammatory markers that can damage the heart and coronary arteries.

VARIATIONS PATHWAYS RELATED TO PROBLEMS WITH THE HEART

Oftentimes, problems with the heart itself, rather than the coronary arteries, indicate that the risk of heart disease has risen. These problems include the following:

- *Nonspecific Changes to the ST Segment on the Electrocardiogram (EKG)*—As electrical currents move through the heart, they produce "movements" that can be seen on an EKG. One of these movements, called the ST segment, occurs at the end of the heartbeat. Potentially harmful changes in the ST segment are visible on an electrocardiogram and are sometimes picked up during a routine physical examination before a crisis or even any symptoms have occurred.
- *Aortic Calcifications*—Deposits consisting of calcium, cholesterol, and other substances may form in the aorta, the large artery that carries freshly oxygenated blood from the heart to the body. This is a sign of atherosclerosis.
- *Chronic Rapid Heartbeat (Tachycardia)*—A heart rate greater than 100 beats per minute is an indication of problems with the heart and predicts higher risk of heart attack.
- *Slow Heart Rate Recovery After a Treadmill Test*—The heart rate, which is deliberately sped up during a treadmill

test, should return to normal within one to two minutes. Any longer than this indicates a slow heart rate recovery and potential trouble.

- *Excessive Heart Rate Variability*—Alternating rapid and slow heart rates increases the risk of sudden death and coronary heart disease.

- *Left Ventricular Hypertrophy*—This is thickening of the muscle of the left ventricle, the chamber that sends blood out of the heart and through the entire body. It may result in poor cardiac output (a less than adequate amount of blood pumped), heart failure, stiffness of the heart, decreased blood supply to the heart muscle, and abnormal electrical activity in the heart.

- *Diastolic Dysfunction*—Stiffness of the heart muscle, with loss of elasticity, predicts coronary heart disease and heart failure.

- *Proliferation/Growth in Arteries and Heart Muscle*—Unwanted growth in the arteries may make them thick, stiff, inelastic, and narrow, which increases blood pressure and arterial disease. If it occurs in the heart, the heart becomes stiff, inelastic, and thick. The heart's ability to contract is eventually reduced, leading to heart failure.

VARIATIONS PATHWAYS RELATED TO OTHER STATES OR DISEASES

A number of seemingly unrelated diseases and states can contribute to coronary heart disease in different ways. These include the following:

- *Age*—As a person ages, the cardiovascular system also ages. Thus, at age fifty-five in men and sixty in women, age becomes an independent risk predictor for heart disease.

- *Being Male*—Heart disease routinely targets males more often than females until menopause, when the risk equalizes.
- *Central Obesity*—This can be measured as the accumulation of excess "belly fat," as a body mass index (BMI) greater than 30, as an increased waist size (greater than 35 inches in women and 40 inches in men), and as an increased waist-to-hip ratio (in women it should be 0.8 or less; in men 1.0 or less). Excess fat can increase the inflammation level in the body, raising the risk of damage to the coronary arteries.
- *Osteoporosis at Menopause*—This indicates that estrogen deficiency has been long-standing. Since estrogen protects against heart disease, a long-standing deficiency means the heart has been at greater risk for a longer than normal period of time.
- *Chronic Cough or Inflammatory Lung Disease*—Chronic bronchitis or asthma, emphysema, bronchiolitis obliterans organizing pneumonia, and other diseases of the respiratory system can raise the inflammatory burden within the arteries.
- *Chronic Infections*—Herpes simplex virus, cytomegalovirus, Epstein-Barr virus, *Haemophilus influenzae* type B, and other organisms that cause chronic infections can lead to increased inflammation and free radical formation. These infections may originate in an isolated part of the body yet increase inflammation levels throughout the body as their by-products spread.
- H. Pylori *Infection*—A bacterium that infects the stomach and small intestines, *H. pylori* can trigger inflammation by irritating the stomach lining.
- *Elevated Serum Estradiol in Men*—A deficiency of male hormones is associated with heart disease. Estradiol (a form of estrogen) is formed by the conversion of male hormones. When estradiol levels rise, it means that many

male hormones are being converted, which can result in deficiency.

- *Urinary Proteomic Risk Predictors*—Analysis of proteins in the urine may detect polypeptides (protein segments) that indicate the presence of specific diseases. More than 238 of these related to coronary heart disease have been identified.

IS THERE A NUMBER-ONE RISK PREDICTOR?

People often ask me which variation or group of variations is most important. I tell them it depends on each person's genetics, biochemistry, and lifestyle. For some people, anger, depression, and other psychological items are the key. I've seen many people who exhibited these kinds of behavior who also had low cholesterol and blood pressure and were not overweight or smokers. Yet they wound up in the ER with crushing chest pain—or worse. On the other hand, I've seen many other patients with serene countenances, plus "safe" cholesterol and blood glucose numbers, whose coronary arteries were weakened by decades of periodontal disease or other chronic inflammatory conditions that were ignored for too long. To put it simply, *any* predictor is the most important one if it's the one that harms your heart.

MORE THAN THE STANDARD MANTRA

Simply understanding that there are many variations that signal risk for coronary heart disease is a big step in the right direction. If you do nothing more than take the lists above to your physician and ask him or her to check several of these items, you'll improve your odds of avoiding heart disease.

Chapter Nine

Eating for Optimal Heart Health

W E'VE KNOWN FOR YEARS that what we eat greatly affects cardiovascular health. And diets designed to protect and improve the health of the heart and blood vessels have been around for what seems like forever. For the longest time, a low-fat, low-cholesterol diet was considered the best approach. But in more recent years, the Mediterranean diet and the DASH diet (Dietary Approaches to Stop Hypertension) took precedence, with results supported by solid scientific research. I endorse either approach, although I believe my own diet, the *Integrative Cardiovascular Disease Prevention Program Diet (ICDPPD)*, which combines the best of both of the aforementioned diets and adds key new understandings about nutrition, is even better. But before I introduce the ICDPPD, let's take a look at the DASH and Mediterranean diets and what they have to offer.

THE DASH AND MEDITERRANEAN DIETS— A LITTLE BACKGROUND

The DASH diet, a sensible, "doable" approach to reducing elevated blood pressure, is the brainchild of the National Heart, Lung, and Blood Institute. In short, when compared to the standard American diet, the DASH diet provides more fiber, calcium, magnesium, and potassium but less saturated fat, refined carbohydrates, sugars, and fats. And it really does reduce high blood pressure. In a study of people with hypertension that compared the effects of the DASH diet to the standard American diet and a similar diet with additional servings of vegetables and fruits, the DASH diet reduced blood pressure the most, and the beneficial effects became obvious sooner. Encouraged, the researchers added sodium restriction to the diet (1,500 to 2,400 milligrams per day), renamed it the DASH II diet, and found that it lowered blood pressure even better than the original DASH.

As for the Mediterranean diet, more than fifty years ago researchers noticed that people who lived on the island of Crete in the Mediterranean Sea had very little heart disease and lived long lives, even though they consumed quite a lot of fat. This didn't make sense in light of the idea prevalent at the time, that fat was the worst thing you could eat. Yet it appeared that for those living in Greece, Italy, southern France, the Middle East, and other Mediterranean areas, fat was a vital part of a healthy diet.

The main fat in the Mediterranean diet is olive oil, which helps lower LDL cholesterol and ward off the oxidation of LDL. But the Mediterranean diet has other elements that are just as important to heart health as olive oil. It's based primarily on plant foods, such as vegetables, fruits, whole grains, and legumes (including chickpeas, used to make hummus). Cheese and yogurt are a daily part of the diet, and small amounts of fish, poultry, and eggs are eaten two to three times per week. Surprisingly, red meat is also eaten, although not more than once a week, and red wine (which is loaded with antioxidants) is taken with meals almost every day. Fresh fruit is the favored dessert, and sweets are limited.

The Mediterranean diet is actually very much like the DASH diet, although sodium is not restricted, olive oil is emphasized, and it probably contains more legumes. Yet both adhere to the same basic principles: eat mostly plant-based foods with lesser amounts of fish, poultry, and eggs and eat very little red meat and few sweets.

Why are both so good for your heart? There are myriad explanations, but they boil down to two major reasons: they provide high levels of antioxidants, which help protect against oxidation (most importantly LDL oxidation), and they help fight inflammation, both of which lie at the root of heart disease. Add to that the cholesterol-lowering effects of olive oil (Mediterranean diet), the blood pressure–lowering effects of sodium restriction (DASH II), and the high fiber content of both, which help fight obesity (you fill up faster while eating lower-calorie foods), and you have a terrific recipe for a healthy cardiovascular system.

While the DASH and Mediterranean diets are excellent foundations for heart health, we've learned more about nutrition and health in the years since they were created. And what's missing from these diets is an understanding of the relationship between human health and our evolutionary heritage. Your genes are 99 percent similar to those of very early human beings, which means your nutritional needs and nutritional-genetic responses are very similar to those of, say, Paleolithic humans. Our ancient ancestors consumed a diet consisting mostly of wild game, fish, eggs, and berries, foods that they hunted, caught, picked, or stole from the nest. Eating these foods helped them flourish. And despite the popular notion that the lives of our ancient ancestors were short and unpleasant, there is strong evidence that they were remarkably healthy, strong boned, and free from the chronic diseases that plague us today. (While it's true that many died young, that was primarily due to injuries, the lack of antibiotics, and other problems we don't face today.)

So while "modern" meat, which comes from grain-fed animals and contains lots of saturated fat, is detrimental, meat from wild animals or animals allowed to eat grass and other natural foods is health-enhancing. It provides calories, key nutrients, and omega-3 fatty acids. It also contains omega-6 fatty acids in the proper 1:2 ratio to the omega-3s. And it's lean—free of the huge amounts of marbled fat found in grain-fed animals that are barely allowed to move around. This "modern meat," especially when it's processed into foods like salami and pastrami, is filled with saturated fat, hormones, additives, and other substances that harm health. But "real" meat that comes from animals given the food they are designed to eat and allowed to move freely over a fair amount of land is perfectly in sync with human health needs.

HOW ICDPPD DIFFERS FROM THE MEDITERRANEAN OR DASH DIETS

My ICDPPD is a compilation of the Mediterranean and DASH diets (a sort of "greatest hits" album of healthy foods), incorporating the great amounts of fruits and vegetables, plus the healthy fats of the former and the sodium restriction of the latter. Then, because human beings evolved to eat "real" meat, the ICDPPD incorporates more lean meat, fish, and wild game than either of the other diets. It also limits the consumption of refined carbohydrates and grains (even whole grains). This may come as a shock to those who are used to the "6–11 servings of grains" recommended by the USDA's Food Guide Pyramid, but grains are simply not foods that our bodies have evolved to consume.

Think about it: Grains (the seeds of wild grass) entered the human diet relatively late in evolutionary terms, not until farming began some ten thousand to twelve thousand years ago. Up until that time, humans could certainly have gathered these seeds and eaten them, but the amounts they actually consumed would have been small, since grains are difficult to collect, chew, and digest. It was only when humans figured out how to grow grains in large amounts and then soak, grind, and cook them that they became a mainstay of the diet. But while our digestive, immune, cardiovascular, and other bodily systems were adept at handling meat, vegetables, and fruits, grains were literally a shock to the system. They necessitated a major genetic adaptation that many of us still haven't managed to achieve. It's quite common to have problems handling the gluten in wheat, for example, which triggers inflammation, allergic reactions, and intestinal damage, all of which hamper nutrient absorption. And, of course, when grains are refined to produce the white flour found in bread, pasta, cookies, pastries, and more, their negative effects on blood glucose, body weight, digestion, and the cardiovascular system are nothing short of an abomination. That's why I recommend that you limit your servings of grains to just one per day, and leave the refined grains out completely.

By combining the best of the Mediterranean diet, the DASH diet, and the diet consumed by our ancient ancestors, I created the ICDPPD, a true cornerstone of cardiovascular health. And as you'll see, the foods that make up the ICDPPD target and help contain each of the five major Fast Track to Heart Disease Pathways.

1. *Inflammation*—The ICDPPD is loaded with foods that help fight inflammation, including cold-water fatty fish (containing omega-3 fatty acids), nuts, seeds, beans, and olive oil. It's also very high in foods containing antioxidants, and when oxidative stress levels go down, so does inflammation. The diet also limits or eliminates some

prime inflammation producers: saturated (animal) fat, polyunsaturated oils (e.g., soy or corn oil), and partially hydrogenated fats (trans fats). And it helps fight obesity, an important cause of inflammation.

2. *Oxidative Stress*—One of the best ways to fight oxidative stress is by eating foods that contain antioxidants and free radical quenchers, such as beta-carotene, vitamins C and E, the mineral selenium, polyphenols, flavonoids, lutein, and lycopene. The ICDPPD provides a wealth of anti-oxidants every day with its six servings of colorful vegetables and four servings of fruit.

3. *Dyslipidemia*—The ICDPPD's recommended fats (mono-unsaturated and omega-3s) help to lower total cholesterol, LDL cholesterol, and triglycerides. The omega-3s can also make the blood "thinner" and less likely to form unwanted clots that could trigger a heart attack or stroke. In addition, the diet's many foods rich in soluble fiber (e.g., beans, strawberries) help bind fats in the intestine and lower the cholesterol level.

4. *High Blood Pressure and Abnormal Blood Flow*—Foods included in the ICDPPD that help lower blood pressure include the omega-3s, potassium-rich foods (e.g., blueberries, peanuts), as well as onions and garlic. The sodium content of the ICDPPD is very low, which is important because large amounts of sodium can cause fluid retention and increase blood pressure. Also, the large amounts of fiber in the diet provided by the vegetables and fruits promote greater feelings of fullness, even though the caloric intake is fairly low. This helps fight obesity, a major cause of high blood pressure.

5. *High Blood Sugar and Insulin Levels*—The ICDPPD severely limits grains and refined carbohydrates, which helps prevent blood sugar spikes and crashes and the

excessive release of insulin. Eating the diet's plentiful high-fiber and high-protein foods also helps control blood sugar and insulin levels.

ELEMENTS OF THE ICDPPD

The ICDPPD isn't a "diet" in the sense that it tells you exactly what to eat at every meal and limits you to those foods in certain amounts. Instead, it offers suggestions as to the number of servings of each food group to take in, as well as serving sizes, and allows you to mix and match them as you like. The foods, servings, and serving sizes are as follows:

Vegetables—6 servings

Serving size: 1 cup raw (chopped), ½ cup cooked, 6 ounces vegetable juice

Suggestions: Eat the most colorful vegetables you can find (dark green, red, purple, orange, and yellow-orange), as they tend to contain the most nutrients. Raw is best, but they can be cooked lightly without added salt or fats. You can substitute vegetable juice for one serving per day, but make sure the juice does not contain sodium.

Fruit—4 servings

Serving size: 1 medium, 1 cup raw (chopped), ½ cup canned (no added sugar), 6 ounces juice

Suggestions: Emphasize those eaten by our ancestors. Mixed berries are best: blueberries, blackberries, strawberries, and raspberries. Eat fresh and raw whenever possible. Substitute fruit juice for no more than one serving of fresh fruit per day.

Protein—2–4 servings

Serving size: 6–8 ounces cooked

Suggestions: Eat cold-water, wild-caught fish, like salmon, cod, mackerel, or tuna (farm-raised fish are low in omega-3s), and/or meat in the form of wild game, wild birds, or range-fed beef, chicken, or turkey. Lean cuts only. Trim the fat; take off the skin before cooking. Bake, broil, or roast; don't fry.

Grains—1 serving

Serving size: 1 cup dry or ½ cup cooked cereal, 1 slice bread, 1 cup cooked brown rice, 1 cup cooked pasta; whole grains only

Suggestions: Eat whole-grain cereals, bread, rice, or pasta with no added sugar or sodium.

Fats—2–3 servings

Serving size: 1 tablespoon oil, 2 tablespoons light salad dressing

Suggestions: Oils should be mostly monounsaturated (olive or canola). Avoid saturated fat, trans fats, and hydrogenated fats.

Dairy—2 servings

Serving size: 1 cup whole milk, buttermilk, or full-fat yogurt; 1-½ ounces low-fat, low-sodium cheese

Suggestions: Full-fat milk, buttermilk, and yogurt are preferred because they contain conjugated linoleic acid (CLA). CLA confers many health benefits, including reducing the risk of heart disease and cancer. While dairy products are good sources of calcium, they can also contain moderate amounts of sodium, so they should be eaten in limited quantities.

Dried Beans, Nuts and Seeds—1–2 servings

Serving size: ½ cup cooked beans, 2 tablespoons seeds, ⅓ cup nuts, 3 ounces tofu (a soybean product)

Suggestions: Avoid canned beans (e.g., baked beans) due to high sodium/sugar content. Choose unsalted mixed nuts or seeds.

Sweets—1 serving weekly

Serving size: 1 small piece of cake, 2 cookies, 1 scoop ice cream

Suggestions: Try to avoid completely. The more you stay away from sweets, the less you will crave them.

Foods to Avoid or Severely Limit

Although there are plenty of kinds of foods you can and should eat on the ICDPPD, you'll need to steer clear of a few things:

Artificial Sweeteners

Avoid sucralose (Splenda), aspartame (Equal, NutraSweet) and saccharin (SugarTwin, Sweet'N Low, Necta Sweet). Okay to use small amounts of raw honey or stevia instead.

Refined Carbohydrates—No more than 1 serving a day or less

Serving size: 1 slice bread, 1 cup cooked pasta

Concerning bread, pasta, white potatoes, white rice, sweets, and similar foods, follow this simple rule: If it's white, do not eat it.

Added Salt

Eat only the sodium that nature put in the food, or use added salt sparingly in the form of potassium chloride.

SAMPLE MENU PLAN

Just so you can see what a day's food intake might look like on the ICDPPD, here's a sample menu:

Breakfast

2 eggs or 4 ounces smoked salmon
1 cup blueberries
1 cup plain full-fat yogurt or one serving of whole-grain cereal
(oat bran, steel-cut oats, or buckwheat (kasha))
1 orange or small grapefruit

Lunch

Garlic Chicken and Veggie Stir-Fry (4 ounces cooked chicken,
1 cup red peppers, 1 cup mushrooms, 1 cup snow peas,
1 cup broccoli, 1 cup spinach, 2 cloves garlic, 2 teaspoon
olive oil)
½ sweet potato
½ cup beans
½ cup brown rice
1 banana or 1 cup mixed berries
1 cup green tea

Snack

Veggie Salad (2 cups spinach, 1 sliced tomato, 2 green onions,
⅓ avocado, 4 teaspoons olive oil vinaigrette)
⅓ cup almonds
1 cup plain, full-fat Greek yogurt

Dinner

4 ounces grilled salmon or 6 ounces wild game or range-fed
chicken
½ cup brown rice
1-½ cups steamed vegetables—carrots, onions, squash
1 cup fresh blueberries

Snack

1 apple with natural peanut butter (no added sugar or sodium)

Just by switching from the standard American diet to the ICDPPD, you will be taking in more fiber, protein, good fats, antioxidants, potassium, magnesium, and other heart-healthy substances than before, even if you take no supplements at all. You'll also be taking in less saturated fat, trans fats, sugar, and other food components that can set you on a Fast Track to Heart Disease Pathway.

How to Cut Back on Sodium Without Cutting Back on Flavor

Substituting herbs and spices for salt can be a delicious way to increase the flavor and appeal of your food while helping you scale back on sodium. Here's a short guide to using herbs and spices in everyday foods.

- *Basil*—Known for its savory presence in Italian foods (especially spaghetti sauce), basil goes well with pasta, chicken, fish, and shellfish.
- *Chili Powder*—This "heated" spice adds a savory bite to stews, soups, Mexican food, and beans. Adding chili powder to brown rice or a stir-fry gives a welcome zing.
- *Cinnamon*—This sweet-tasting spice contains no sugar, but you'd never know it. Use it over cereal, with fruit, or as a major ingredient in tea. You'll find you don't need sugar to enjoy sweetness.
- *Curry Powder*—A key ingredient in Indian and Southeast Asian cuisine, curry adds an exotic aroma to steamed vegetables or mashed potatoes.

- *Dill Weed*—Used often in Scandinavian cooking, dill goes beautifully with fish, vegetables, poultry, and yogurt. Mix 1 teaspoon dill weed with 2 tablespoons trans-fat-free margarine. Spread on vegetables and heat until melted.
- *Mint*—This delightfully fresh tasting leaf can be chopped and sprinkled over sliced fruit or cooked peas or used as a garnish for fish, poultry, or meat dishes.
- *Nutmeg*—Instantly recognizable as the garnish used for eggnog, nutmeg's inherent sweetness complements cooked carrots, fresh fruit, ground meat, and yogurt.
- *Rosemary*—This savory herb is a natural for poultry, meats, roasted vegetables, and water-sautéed mushrooms. It also tastes terrific with ripe melon.
- *Tarragon*—This herb, which tastes somewhat like licorice, goes well with fish, poultry, shellfish, and eggs, as well as tomatoes, carrots, and mushrooms. It's particularly delicious when added to vinaigrette salad dressings.
- *Turmeric*—This essential ingredient of most curries gives Indian food its earthy, savory taste. It also adds color and taste to light-yellow vegetables, such as squash.

WEIGHT LOSS AND THE INTEGRATIVE CARDIOVASCULAR DISEASE PREVENTION PROGRAM DIET

My ICDPPD isn't intended to be a weight-loss diet, but slimming down to your optimal weight and body fat percentage is vitally important to the health of your heart. If you are overweight or obese, losing weight has endless health advantages, including reducing:

- the amount of inflammation-producing fat packed around the belly
- the risk of insulin resistance
- the risk of metabolic syndrome
- the risk of diabetes, which harms the lining of the blood vessels
- the factors that increase blood pressure and oxidative stress and cause "bad" cholesterol numbers

How do you know if you need to lose weight? The best way to find out is to have your body-fat percentage measured by your doctor or physical therapist. You can get a fairly good idea on your own simply by calculating your body mass index, or BMI. Just divide your body weight (in kilograms) by your height (in meters) squared.

If you prefer to use the more familiar pounds and inches:

1. Multiply your weight in pounds by 0.45 (i.e., if you weigh 120 pounds, multiply 120 by 0.45 to get 54).
2. Multiply your height in inches by 0.025 (i.e., if you're 5 feet 4 inches, you're 64 inches tall. 64 x 0.025 = 1.6).
3. Multiply your answer from step 2 by itself (i.e., 1.6 x 1.6 = 2.56).
4. Divide your answer from step 1 by your answer from step 3 (i.e., 54 / 2.56 = 21.09, which rounds off to 21).

Your BMI is 21.

Using myself as an example, here's how I can use that formula to find my BMI:

1. Multiply my weight in pounds, 195, by 0.45 to get 87.75.
2. Multiply my height in inches, 73, by 0.025 to get 1.825.
3. Multiply 1.825 by itself to get 3.33.
4. Divide 87.75 by 3.33 to get 26.35.

My BMI is 26.35.

Once you've calculated your BMI, you can easily see where you stand: a BMI less than 25 is normal, 25–30 is overweight, and over 30 indicates obesity. This BMI calculation doesn't work well for people who are well muscled, like football players, as their extra poundage is "good" weight, not fat. Neither does it work well for models or other people who are exceptionally skinny, for they may weigh so little due to a lack of muscle mass and thinning bones, although they may still carry relatively large amounts of fatty tissue. For most people, however, the BMI is a good rough guide. (Even better is to have body fat and lean muscle mass measured via body impedance analysis, which works by measuring the resistance electrical currents meet as they run through the body. Electricity moves more easily through water than through fat, and muscle contains more water than does fat. The easier it is for electricity to move from one specified point in the body to another, the more muscle and less fat there is.)

If you need to lose weight, you can adjust your daily caloric intake downward by eating smaller amounts of the recommended servings from each group.

IT ALL BEGINS WITH ONE STEP

If following this diet sounds difficult, don't worry. You don't have to become a perfect "lean, mean eating machine" overnight. Think of the ICDPPD as being the goalposts at the end of the football field. Keep moving in that direction, no matter how long it takes to get there and no matter how many times you're "tackled" by salty, fatty, or processed foods.

Begin by increasing your servings of fruits and vegetables while reducing refined carbohydrates (the white foods), sweets, and grains and lowering your saturated and trans fat intake. Stop consuming all forms of soda. Gradually cut back on your

Servings Per Day

	Grains	Vegetables	Fruits	Whole milk and milk products	Lean meats, poultry, and fish	Nuts, seeds, and legumes	Fats and oils	Sweets and added sugars
1,600 calories per day	1	6	4	2	2–4	1–2	2–3	0–1
2,600 calories per day	1–2	8	4	4	5	2	3–4	2 or less
3,100 calories per day	1–2	10	4	4	7	2	4–5	2 or less

salt, but not to the point where your food is tasteless. You'll probably find that your food is actually tastier once you ease up on the salt and that fresh fruits and vegetables have subtle but delicious flavors that you weren't aware of in the past. Do the best you can, but if you slip up and eat an "unapproved" meal once in a while, don't worry. Pick up where you left off, and make sure your next meal puts you back on track. Remember that heart-healthy eating is a marathon, not a sprint.

RECIPES

To help you get started on your new eating plan, here are a few examples of some delicious, heart-healthy, blood pressure–lowering recipes. The recipes are adapted from recipes offered by the Centers for Disease Control and Prevention (http://apps.nccd.cdc.gov/dnparecipe/recipesearch.aspx) and conform to the principles of my ICDPPD. Try them as is, or use them for inspiration when making up your own recipes.

Breakfast Ideas

Golden Apple Oatmeal

Preparation Time: 15 minutes
Number of Servings: 1

1 Golden Delicious apple, diced
⅔ cup water
Dash of cinnamon
Dash of nutmeg
⅓ cup quick-cooking rolled oats, uncooked

Combine apples, water, and seasonings; bring to a boil. Stir in oats; cook 3–5 minutes. Cover and let stand several minutes before serving.

Swiss Muesli

Preparation Time: 20 minutes
Number of Servings: 3

¾ cup rolled oats
¾ cup water
1 cup shredded, unpeeled apples
1 dried fig
1 tablespoon lemon juice
¼ teaspoon cinnamon
¼ cup chopped almonds
1 tablespoon ground flaxseed

Combine oats, water, shredded apples, dried fig lemon juice, cinnamon, chopped almonds, and flaxseed. Cover and refrigerate overnight. In the morning, spoon some of the muesli into a cereal bowl. Top with your choice of fresh fruits and nuts. Serve with a dollop of plain yogurt or almond milk, if desired. Muesli can be stored in a covered container in the refrigerator for several days.

Black and Blue Berry Smoothie

Smoothies are a quick and easy way to ensure a healthy breakfast. This recipe and the one that follows are loaded with beta-carotene, protein, flavonoids, pectin, and vitamin C. Try frozen strawberries, blueberries, mixed berries, mango, or peaches. If you add juice, you might try pineapple juice, orange-tangerine juice, and other 100-percent juice blends.

Preparation Time: 10 minutes
Number of Servings: 2

1 scoop whey protein powder (look for one with about 20 grams protein per serving)

½ cup blackberries
½ cup blueberries
½ cup full-fat plain yogurt
½ cup organic whole milk
½ teaspoon vanilla extract
1 cup ice

Place all ingredients into blender and blend until smooth. Serve immediately.

Raspberry Mango Smoothie

Preparation Time: 5 minutes
Number of Servings: 1

1 cup unsweetened, frozen raspberries
1 scoop vanilla whey protein powder
1 cup almond milk
5 ice cubes
1 teaspoon cinnamon

Blend well in blender and serve.

Salads as a Side Dish

Jicama and Asian Pear Salad

Preparation Time: 15 minutes
Number of Servings: 6

2 cups shredded romaine lettuce
2 cups julienned jicama
2 cored and chopped Asian pears
1 tablespoon golden raisins
¼ cup white wine vinaigrette salad dressing

¼ cup apple cider vinegar
¼ teaspoon Chinese five-spice powder or ground allspice

In a bowl, toss the shredded lettuce, jicama, Asian pears, and golden raisins until combined. For dressing, whisk together the salad dressing, apple cider vinegar, and spice until well mixed. Drizzle over salad and toss well. Serve immediately.

Pineapple Slaw

Preparation Time: 10 minutes
Number of Servings: 6

2-½ cups shredded cabbage
1 cup shredded carrots
1 cup pineapple chunks
1 tablespoon raisins
2-½ tablespoons pineapple juice
1 tablespoon olive or grape seed oil

Combine all ingredients in a large bowl. Toss and serve, or put in refrigerator, covered, until serving time.

Apple-Hazelnut Salad in a Cup

Preparation Time: 10 minutes
Number of Servings: 1

2 tablespoons nonfat bottled raspberry vinaigrette
1 diced apple
2 tablespoons chopped hazelnuts
1 cup precut mixed greens, rinsed and drained

Layer ingredients in order, with dressing on the bottom, in a large, travel-proof, lidded, insulated cup. When ready to eat, shake the cup well, grab a fork, and enjoy!

Entrees

Lentil Soup—Indian Style

Preparation Time: 2 hours
Number of Servings: 8

1 pound dry lentils, picked over and rinsed
10 cups water
2 onions, chopped
1 green pepper, chopped
2 cloves garlic, finely minced
2 teaspoon salt
½ teaspoon black pepper
1 15-ounce can low-sodium tomato sauce
½ teaspoon cinnamon
2 cardamom pods
1 teaspoon turmeric
1 teaspoon coriander
⅜ teaspoon crushed red pepper flakes
2 teaspoons curry powder

Combine lentils and water with onion, green pepper, garlic, salt, and pepper. Bring to a boil and simmer 30 minutes.

Add other ingredients; simmer 1 hour. Strain out cardamom pods. Blend about three-quarters of the soup in a blender. Return blended soup to pot and stir.

Salmon Tacos

Preparation Time: 30 minutes
Number of Servings: 6

½ cup sour cream
¼ cup mayonnaise

½ cup chopped fresh cilantro
½ package low-sodium taco seasoning, divided
1 pound salmon (or cod) fillets, cut into 1-inch pieces
1 tablespoon olive oil
2 tablespoons lemon juice
2 cups shredded red and green cabbage
2 cups diced tomato
12 6-inch warmed Trader Joe's (or other organic) low-carbohydrate wheat tortillas
Lime wedges for serving
Low-sodium taco sauce for seasoning

In a small bowl, combine sour cream, mayonnaise, cilantro, and 2 tablespoons of the seasoning mix. In medium bowl, combine salmon, olive oil, lemon juice, and remaining seasoning mix; pour into large skillet. Cook, stirring constantly, over medium-high heat for 4 to 5 minutes, or until salmon flakes easily when tested with a fork. Fill warm tortillas with fish mixture. Top with cabbage, tomato, sour cream mixture, lime wedges, and taco sauce.

Tuna-Bean Main Dish Salad

Preparation Time: 4 hours, 15 minutes
Number of Servings: 6

Dressing

½ teaspoon grated lemon peel
⅓ cup lemon juice
¼ cup olive oil
2 tablespoons fresh chopped parsley
1 teaspoon rosemary
1 tablespoon Dijon mustard

Mix all ingredients thoroughly and store in a tightly covered container in the refrigerator until ready to be used.

Salad

3 medium green bell peppers
3 medium red bell peppers
2 15-ounce cans white beans, rinsed and drained
2 6-ounce cans low-sodium, water-packed tuna, drained
½ cup sliced ripe olives
1 head lettuce
2 medium tomatoes, cut into wedges

Set oven to broil. Place bell peppers on broiler pan. Broil with tops 4 to 5 inches from heat, about 3–5 minutes on each side or until skin blisters and browns. Remove from oven. Wrap in towel; let stand 5 minutes. Remove skin, stems, seeds, and membranes of the peppers. Cut peppers into ¼-inch slices. Toss peppers, beans, tuna, olives, and dressing in a bowl. Cover and chill for 4 hours, stirring occasionally. Spoon salad onto lettuce leaves and garnish with tomato wedges.

Lasagna

Preparation Time: 1 hour, 30 minutes
Number of Servings: 9

1 pound ground, range-fed turkey
1 pound cottage cheese
½ pound ricotta cheese
2 egg whites
1 tablespoon grated low-fat Parmesan cheese
1 tablespoon fresh minced chives
1 tablespoon fresh minced parsley
¼ teaspoon freshly ground black pepper
8 ounces whole wheat lasagna noodles, uncooked

1 large onion, minced
¼ cup dry red wine
½ pound sliced mushrooms
1 cup chopped zucchini
4 cups low-sodium tomato sauce of your choice

In a nonstick frying pan, cook ground turkey until it is no longer pink; drain juices and set aside.

Puree cottage cheese, ricotta, egg whites, and Parmesan cheese in blender. Blend in chives, parsley, and pepper by hand.

In a large pot of lightly salted boiling water, cook lasagna noodles until just tender but not mushy, about 10 minutes. Remove noodles with a slotted spoon, dip into cold water, and lay out flat on clean kitchen towels (not paper towels, or they will stick).

In covered skillet, simmer onions in wine for about 5 minutes, or until very soft. Stir frequently, but keep pot covered between stirrings. Add mushrooms and zucchini and cook about 5 minutes, or until vegetables are soft and half their original volume. Drain the vegetables.

Preheat oven to 375°F. Combine the cheese mixture and all but ¼ cup of the vegetable mixture. Spread 2 cups tomato sauce over the bottom of a 9- by 14-inch baking pan. Alternate layers of noodles with cheese mixture and ground turkey, ending with a final layer of noodles. Cover noodles with remaining sauce, and distribute reserved vegetables over the top.

Cover and bake for 1 hour. Remove cover and bake for an additional 5 minutes. Remove from oven and let the lasagna sit for 10 minutes before cutting.

Chapter Ten

ABCT Exercise: The Theory

THERE IS A SECRET about cardiovascular health that most physicians do not know: Specific kinds of exercise can alter the ways genes function and interact with your cells. By triggering the right exercise-gene interactions, you can tamp down inflammation, reduce oxidation, strengthen your cardiovascular system, turn your body into a fat-burning machine, and slow—or even reverse—many aspects of aging.

The slow physical deterioration of the arteries and other body parts we typically see with age is *not* inevitable. It is largely the result of diet and movement—or the lack thereof. Movement is one of the primary keys to cardiovascular health, but not just any type of movement will do. Doing a thousand sit-ups, jogging 10 miles, or practicing yoga every day won't do the trick. The movement your need is the same kind of natural movement that kept humans in robust physical health for millennia. This is not the kind of exercise that most personal trainers, fitness enthusiasts, or doctors recommend. As a matter of fact, most doctors and trainers recommend the exact *opposite* approach to movement and exercise, one that may actually accelerate deterioration of the arteries and encourage overall aging.

The problem lies in the fact that to the average exerciser, trainer, and physician, exercise is all about working the heart and lungs while burning off calories. But the power of exercise goes well beyond that, for as muscles move, they release powerful messenger molecules that "speak" to every organ in the body and determine whether oxidation and inflammation are encouraged or discouraged, fat is burned or stored, new tissue is created, and much more.

A LITTLE BIOCHEMICAL BACKGROUND

Most people think of genes as being the brains of a cell. They believe that unless the genes constantly tell the cell what to do, it will die. But if you remove the genes from a cell, it goes right on living: synthesizing energy, eliminating wastes, and behaving like any other cell. Rather than being the brains of the cell, the genes are more like the fix-it manual. When a worn-out part of a cell needs to be replaced or new substances need to be created from scratch, the genes provide instructions for doing so.

Genes are the individual units in the long sequence of genetic material tucked into each and every cell in the body. Think of this genetic material as a huge instruction manual. The genetic material can be read by the cells only when the manual is opened to the proper page—in other words, the right gene. This is indeed what happens, for the genetic fix-it manual is regularly opened to a specific page so the instructions can be read, then closed, then opened again to a new page, and so on. But this opening and closing doesn't happen randomly; it occurs only when the cell needs to read a particular piece of genetic code. That happens on a routine basis, as the cell needs more of this or that substance for everyday purposes. It also happens, quite often, in response to messages sent from other parts of the body. The messengers tell the cell which "pages" need to be read by "plugging into" the cell membrane.

Every cell is surrounded by a membrane that is studded with thousands of receptors. These receptors receive information coming from other parts of the body, passing it into the cell, where it is acted on: specific proteins are made, more or fewer calories are burned, and so on. The receptor-covered membrane is the cell's command center, or brain. If you remove these receptors from the cell membrane, the cell goes comatose and soon dies (even though the genes are intact).

The fact that a cell cannot survive without its receptors underscores the fact that the cell's function is largely controlled by factors outside the cell—specifically, by the hormones and other messenger molecules that bind to the membrane receptors and tell the cell what to do.

These messengers are not randomly generated by the body. They are created in response to what is happening inside and outside the body. This means your lifestyle, diet, thoughts and behaviors, the temperature, light and sounds you are exposed to, and especially your movement and exercise determine which messages are sent, and therefore which genes are activated and which are left quiet. You may have been born with some defective genes—perhaps some that increase the risk of developing breast cancer—but it is often the messengers produced by your environmental choices that determine whether or not those genes are activated.

Genes may enhance or limit a cell's ability to respond to messages and create substances, but it's the hormones and other messengers that drive the cellular action by issuing the orders.

MUSCLE MOLECULES ARE THE KEY

A hormone is a substance produced in one part of the body that travels to another part to trigger a desired action, with the action depending on which hormone is sent and where. The body produces many different hormones, including testosterone, estrogen, progesterone, cortisol, insulin, growth hormone, adrenaline, and DHEA.

Hormones have numerous functions in the body. For example, they control fuel mechanisms, determining not only how many calories to burn but also what type of fuel to use (sugar or fat) and where to take that fuel from (arms, legs, belly, etc.). They also impact reproduction, hunger, immune function, and every other metabolic process in the body—even the way genes are expressed ("read" and used). Controlling the hormones means controlling the body. And a powerful way to do that is through movement.

Human physiology is designed around movement, with several different hormones being released by body movement. Different kinds of movement send different hormonal signals, which attach to receptors on the membranes of different cells. Unfortunately, most of us don't move nearly enough, and when we do, it's usually the wrong way, which either doesn't produce the health-enhancing message we'd like or actually produces "antihealth" messages that spread throughout the body.

EXERCISING TO TRIGGER GOOD STRESS

Most people exercise to lose weight. That's commendable but a waste of time, for exercise is not about burning calories. This focus on caloric expenditure is the sole reason that so many people fail to attain, or fail to maintain, better bodies with exercise. Exercise is really about genetic signaling via hormones. But not all exercise has the same effect on genetic signaling.

Think about muscular Olympic sprinters and wiry and gaunt Olympic marathon runners. Both have low percentages of body fat, but the sprinters have even less. That sounds odd, for marathon runners burn many more calories than sprinters while running incredibly long distances. The key difference is that sprinters exercise in very short, all-out bursts of energy, while marathon runners exercise for hours at a slower, steadier pace.

Caloric expenditure is really just a side effect of exercise, inconsequential compared to the huge release of hormones and other signaling substances that drive body function. While the short, intense activity of sprinting does not burn many calories, it triggers the release of adrenaline, human growth hormone, cortisol, and testosterone. This hormonal mix elevates caloric consumption for hours and even days after the sprinter has stopped running. Long-distance running does not elicit the same effect. Instead, it leads to the production of a different hormonal mix that causes muscle wasting, inefficient metabolic processing, and physical decay.

SOME KEY MOLECULES OF "MUSCLE TALK"

Whether you are sitting still in your chair, playing softball, running a marathon, or lifting weights, your muscles are constantly talking with the rest of the body via the signals they send out to the brain, liver, fat cells, and other tissues. What the muscles are "saying" depends on what you're doing. Higher-intensity exercise gets the muscles talking the most. Exercise using full body movements, incorporating great amounts of muscle, requiring a combination of strength and endurance, and forcing the muscles to do a lot of work in a little bit of time causes the muscles to shout out a unique message that sets in motion a powerful muscle-building, fat-burning, anti-inflammatory, and brain-stimulating effect. Let's take a quick look at some of the more potent of these substances released by movement and exercise.

Interleukin-6 (IL-6)—Fat Burning and Inflammation Control

IL-6 informs the body about the muscle's current and future energy needs. The most powerful metabolic signaling agent released from muscle, it is sent out as soon as muscle starts to contract and move. It's released in even greater amounts as the activity becomes more intense. IL-6's actions help dampen inflammation, raise levels of testosterone and growth hormone, increase fat burning, regulate glucose, reduce weight, increase muscle mass, fine-tune fuel metabolism, and reduce the risk of heart disease and stroke.

Interleukin-15 (IL-15)—Muscle Sparing and Fat Burning

The major task of IL-15, which is released primarily through weight training, is to regulate the breakdown of muscle tissue. It is a major factor in determining the body's muscle-to-fat ratio, which is an important contributor to coronary heart disease and one of the first things to change for the worse with age. Unfortunately, most modern exercise regimens do not trigger the release of adequate amounts of IL-15, for they avoid the short bursts of intense energy expenditure needed to produce it in sufficient amounts.

Interleukin-8 (IL-8)—Making New Blood Vessels

IL-8 is synthesized in muscle whenever the muscle is forced to produce energy without oxygen. When this happens, the muscle releases IL-8, which calls for new blood vessels to grow so the muscle can get enough fresh oxygen the next time around. This is a remarkable example of exercise's ability to mold metabolism. As the muscle talks to the rest of the body, it sets into motion a set of instructions that make it more efficient, leaner, and younger.

Lactic Acid—Growth Promoter, Energy Enhancer

Lactic acid, also known as lactate, used to be considered a waste product. Today we understand that it really has several beneficial effects. One of the immediate effects of lactic acid is to balance out the great deal of acidity that builds up as a result of intense movement. The burn you feel during intense exercise, usually blamed on lactic acid, is really caused by the buildup of toxic metabolic waste products, such as ammonia and hydrogen. Lactic acid buffers their effects and allows the body to perform better for longer.

New research has shown that lactic acid circulating through the blood behaves like a hormone, stimulating the release of testosterone and growth hormone, two powerful growth promoters that make the whole body stronger, leaner, and more functional. In addition, lactic acid signals the muscle cells to increase the number of energy factories (mitochondria) within the cells, meaning the body can burn more fat to produce more energy and support bodily functions.

Unfortunately, getting to the state where lactic acid is released is uncomfortable, and most people avoid it like the plague, opting for slower and lower-intensity forms of exercise, like jogging or peddling a bike. But only intense bursts of activity that trigger "the burn" can get the muscles talking to the rest of the body and forcing it to adapt and grow.

Nitric Oxide—The Blood Flow Effect

Blood is the body's lifeline, and nitric oxide is a major factor in regulating blood flow. Nitric oxide has numerous beneficial effects, including reducing arterial inflammation, lowering oxidative stress throughout the body, opening the arteries wider, inhibiting thickening of the arteries, decreasing atherosclerosis, lowering blood pressure, and reducing blood clotting and platelet stickiness.

It has traditionally been thought that nitric oxide production is largely controlled by the endothelial cells. We've learned, however, that activated muscles also release this powerful molecule, allowing blood vessels supplying the muscle to remain open and keep valuable blood flowing to the area. Being able to harness the effects of nitric oxide through muscle action opens up a powerful pathway for improving the activity of blood vessels, as well as regulating blood pressure and influencing coronary heart disease and other ailments of the blood vessels.

ABCT EXERCISE

In the next chapter, I'll describe my ABCT Exercise Program, a modern way of exercising the way our ancestors did. The program is specifically designed to get your muscles and body moving in short bursts of intense activity, mixing anaerobic with just enough aerobic exercise to improve your arteries and heart health—as well as your overall conditioning.

The ABCT Exercise Program has numerous positive effects on body and mind, much more than the typical aerobic-based programs. Among other things, it:

- reduces risk of heart disease and heart attack and lowers risk of recurrent heart attack
- improves heart function
- lowers blood pressure and reduces risk of developing hypertension
- reduces total cholesterol, triglycerides, and LDL
- increases HDL
- reduces body weight and body fat
- reduces clotting tendencies
- lowers blood sugar and decreases risk of diabetes
- improves insulin sensitivity
- improves all abnormalities of metabolic syndrome
- improves immune function
- reduces risk of stroke

- reduces risk of certain cancers, such as colon, breast, and prostate
- improves memory and focus and reduces risk of Alzheimer's disease and dementia
- improves skin tone and elasticity and decreases wrinkles
- improves depression, stress, anxiety, and overall psychological well-being
- improves sleep

It's easy to get started and simple to follow, so let's begin.

Chapter Eleven

ABCT Exercise: The Practice

You are about to embark on a revolutionary exercise program that will change your life and improve your health beyond your wildest dreams. My ABCT Exercise Program is simple, effective, scientifically proven, and adaptable to everyone's exercise needs. It allows you to enjoy optimal training benefits in a shorter period of time, build and tone muscle, reduce body fat, lose weight, improve hormone levels, lower inflammation and oxidation, decrease blood sugar, reduce blood pressure, and push down LDL while increasing HDL. In addition to reducing your risk of developing coronary heart disease, the ABCT Exercise Program lowers your risk of suffering stroke, diabetes, metabolic syndrome, insulin resistance, Alzheimer's disease, dementia, and cancer while improving your quality of life and increasing your life expectancy. It can even slow the aging process—literally.

THE ABCS OF EXERCISE WITH A TWIST

The most efficient and effective means of achieving all the health benefits of exercise is to combine interval aerobic with anaerobic or resistance exercise in a way that causes the body to kick into restoration and growth overdrive. My ABCT Exercise Program does just that. ABCT stands for Aerobics, Build, Contour, and Tone. It has additional meanings that help define its goals:

- *A* = *Aerobics*, plus *action* and *adaptation*—The program focuses on the types of action best suited for muscle and cardiovascular conditioning. You will adapt to new exercises so your muscles do not accommodate or become "used to" the same daily training.

- *B* = *Build*, plus *bulk*, *burn*, and *breathe*—The program builds and increases muscle strength more than any other exercise regimen you have tried before. (Males will build bulk, while women generally do not increase bulk but will instead tone, firm, and sculpt, due to hormonal differences.) You'll use the muscle burn to the best advantage. And with proper breathing, you'll increase oxygen consumption while removing carbon dioxide to improve cardiovascular and muscle conditioning and function while reducing fatigue.

- *C* = *Contour*, plus *core* and *controlling your genes*—Muscular exercise regulates the expression of more than four hundred genes that mediate the beneficial effects of physical activity. In addition to aerobics and resistance exercise, you will practice core exercises that improve abdominal and back muscle strength while increasing flexibility and balance.

- *T* = *Tone*, plus *trim* and *tight*—You will trim away total fat as well as central or visceral body fat, lose weight, and increase your lean muscle mass. Your muscles, subcutaneous tissue, and skin will become tight and look more youthful.

A FEW WORDS OF CAUTION

The ABCT Exercise Program emphasizes interval aerobic and anaerobic resistance movements, but do not overlook the importance of warming up and stretching before beginning every exercise session and of cooling down and stretching again when you are finished. Doing so will help you avoid muscle, tendon, and ligament injuries while promoting the flexibility that's necessary for exercising and all of your other activities.

Before embarking on an exercise program of any kind or changing the exercise regimen you already have, consult with your personal physician. It's important to ensure that your heart and cardiovascular system are healthy enough to allow you to exercise safely. In addition, interval training with rapid bursts of activity may precipitate plaque rupture in a coronary artery in some predisposed individuals and result in a coronary clot and heart attack. Every patient who plans on doing an interval training program should have a complete cardiovascular exam that includes an exercise treadmill test, physical exam, history, and assessment of cardiac risk factors prior to doing this type of exercise.

THE ELEMENTS OF ABCT

Here are the main elements of ABCT, each of which will be discussed in more detail later.

- *Resistance Training*—Weight lifting modified to spur the muscles to "talk" to the body in such a way as to encourage better heart and full-body health. ABCT uses graduated weights and variable repetitions. In brief, lift the heaviest weight you can twelve times to get the burn, then decrease the weight with each subsequent set—but keep increasing the number of times you lift that weight. This maximizes postexercise oxygen consumption, depletes glycogen, and increases the production of lactic acid to achieve all the muscle-, hormone-, cytokine-, and interleukin-stimulating effects that lead to the health benefits of exercise.

- *Aerobic Training in Intervals*—Jogging, swimming, and other forms of continual movement set the heart beating at an elevated rate and keep it there for a predetermined amount of time. However, the standard approach—keeping the heart beating at a certain elevated rate for twenty, thirty, or even sixty minutes—is faulty. The best technique is aerobic interval training, which consists of short periods ranging from twenty seconds to two minutes of "burst" aerobic training of varying intensities, depending on your present level of exercise conditioning. This more closely mimics the natural activities we evolved to perform and benefit from and strings together several periods of intense and semi-intense activity into a single, longer exercise period that still burns calories and builds endurance.

- *Proper Ratio of Aerobic Training to Resistance Training*— The optimal ratio of resistance to interval aerobic training should be 2:1. For example, during a sixty-minute workout, you would perform forty minutes of resistance training and twenty minutes of interval aerobics, with the aerobics coming after the resistance training.

- *Core Exercises*—Exercises designed to improve abdominal and back strength while increasing flexibility. These exercises are important for the core (abdomen and lower back), which is often neglected and not nearly strong enough in most people.

- *Time-Intense Exercise*—Rather than methodically working one muscle or muscle group after another, then doing the aerobic exercises—or even saving the aerobics for the next day—ABCT challenges the body by combining exercises as much as possible. For example, instead of doing leg squats followed by shoulder presses, with ABCT they are done at the same time, mimicking the real-life movements our bodies were designed to thrive on.

- *Busy Rest Periods*—These are used to insert small bursts of aerobic exercises into the resistance training period.
- *Water and the ABCT Energy Shake*—Drinking plenty of water while working out is vital. (If you get thirsty during the workout, you have waited too long to drink.) You must drink water before beginning to exercise, at set intervals during exercise, and afterwards. Your water should be of high quality and *not* from plastic containers, due to the risk of certain chemical compounds that get into the water from the plastic. In addition, about ten minutes after starting your workout, you begin drinking a special ABCT Energy Shake consisting of fresh orange juice and water, raw honey, d-ribose, carnitine, glutamine, vitamin C, and whey protein to provide energy and nutritional substrates to maximize exercise performance and build muscle.
- *Morning Exercise*—Exercising in the morning after a twelve-hour fast is best for numerous reasons, including the fact that an empty stomach optimizes fat burning, IL-6 and myokine surges, resulting in an increase in muscle strength, bulk, tone and contour, as well as weight loss. In addition, you will be more energized during the rest of the day and enjoy enhanced focus and concentration.
- *Fasting Exercise*—Begin exercising on an empty stomach after a twelve-hour fast, except for water and whey protein consumed about ten minutes before exercise, and have nothing but more water and the ABCT Energy Shake while exercising. This allows for depletion of liver and muscle glycogen while generating maximal surges of IL-6. It also increases fat burning and accelerates weight and fat loss from both inside and outside the muscle.
- *Push and Rest*—Exercise to maximal effort during each set, pushing until "the burn" is significant. The burn

should be severe and last for about four to five seconds after you stop the exercise. You should then rest for sixty seconds before beginning the next set or exercise and may take three-second rest periods between repetitions, if necessary. You can also perform supersets with minimal rest between sets of exercises or use the rest period for core exercises or alternative upper or lower body exercises to improve the time intensity of your exercise session.

- *Daily Exercise, Utilizing Cross-Training*—Perform interval aerobic and resistance training every day to achieve the best results. Do different kinds of exercise to utilize more muscle groups and reduce the risk of injury.
- *Proper Breathing*—Mastering proper breathing techniques will ensure ample supplies of oxygen for the muscles, as well as prompt removal of carbon dioxide.

THE ABCT ELEMENTS, IN DEPTH

Now let's take a look at each of the elements.

Resistance Training

You're undoubtedly familiar with resistance training, which involves lifting weights, doing push-ups, and so on. People who perform resistance training are usually interested in bulking up, getting larger and "ripped" muscles, or toning and contouring their muscles without making them too large. Generally speaking, those interested in bulking up perform fewer lifts with heavier weights, while those who prefer to tone and contour lift lighter weights more times.

ABCT Resistance Training takes a radically different approach, mixing heavier weights and lower repetitions with lower weights and greater repetitions to increase the lactic acid burn as well as to maximize muscle contractions and the release of myokines. With ABCT, the real goal is neither to bulk nor to contour the muscles but to use muscle movements to improve body biochemistry. (Your muscles will certainly become stronger with ABCT, and you can do additional lifts to sculpt the look you prefer.)

ABCT Resistance Training is based on five sets, each with a different number of repetitions. (A repetition is a single lift; a set is a group of repetitions done together.) It starts with the heaviest weight you can handle for one set and works down and then back up from there. When you're done, you feel as if you couldn't do another lift at that weight. Here's the ABCT Five-Set Schedule.

- ABCT Set 1: 12 repetitions at maximum weight
- ABCT Set 2: 18 repetitions at 75 percent of maximum weight
- ABCT Set 3: 24 repetitions at 50 percent of maximum weight
- ABCT Set 4: 50 repetitions at 25 percent of maximum weight
- ABCT Set 5: 12 repetitions at maximum weight

It's difficult to jump right into the ABCT Five-Set schedule, so it's okay to begin slowly and work your way into it, depending on your present level of physical conditioning.

- Beginner: ABCT 1, or ABCT 1 and 2
- Intermediate: ABCT 1, 2, and 3
- Advanced: ABCT 1, 2, 3, and 4
- Professional: ABCT 1, 2, 3, 4, and 5

Don't be alarmed by the title "Professional." Anyone can build up to it; it just takes time and discipline.

Use this Burn Scale as a guide to how hard you should be

working. The idea is to attempt to score a 5 multiple times during your workouts, stopping only briefly (three seconds) to clear the burn before continuing again.

1—No burn in the muscle
2—Light burn
3—Moderate burn
4—Strong burn
5—Intense burn; must rest

What, How, and When to Lift

You'll find descriptions of the key ABCT resistance exercises at the end of the chapter under the heading "Getting Started with ABCT: Training Schedules and Descriptions of the Lifts."

Upping the Intensity with Supersets, Hybrids, and Rapid Sets

Simply following the ABCT Five-Set Schedule will help improve your cardiovascular and general health. But you can do even more for your health by incorporating hybrids, supersets, and rapid sets as you gain strength and endurance.

- *Hybrids* are two exercises performed at once; that is, doing a full leg squat while also performing an overhead press. Using more muscles simultaneously increases the burn, lactic acid, release of IL-6, and postexercise oxygen consumption.
- *Supersets* are exercises done back to back, with almost no rest period between (fifteen seconds maximum). These can be the same exercise, such as biceps curls back to back, or different exercises, such as a biceps curl followed immediately by a triceps lift. Supersets dramatically increase the burn and other beneficial effects of exercise. Supersets should be done only after you have trained

for some time to avoid overuse injury or excessive heart rate.

- *Rapid sets* are sets performed faster than normal to compress the workout time, enhance mechanical and metabolic burnout, and improve both resistance and aerobic conditioning. For example, if you are doing a biceps curl, you can increase the speed from one every second to two every three seconds.

Hybrids, supersets, and rapid sets can do wonders for your cardiovascular and general health, but they can be harmful if you're not prepared to do them. Don't attempt any of these more intense exercises until you've mastered the basic ABCT exercises and can push yourself without harm.

ABCT Resistance Training Hints

1. Take three-second breaks along the way, if necessary.
2. Drink water and the ABCT Energy Shake after each set of exercises.
3. If you cannot do the required number of repetitions in any set, don't worry. Just push as hard as you can until you get the maximum burn.
4. If the percentage reduction in weight is a fraction of a number, round up to the next highest whole number on the weight system you are using. For example, if you started with 25 pounds as your maximal weight, then 75 percent would be 18.75 pounds, which means you would wind up using a 20-pound weight. The 50-percent level is 12.5 pounds, so round up to 15 pounds.

Aerobic Training in Intervals

Aerobic means "with oxygen" and refers to the use of oxygen in the body's metabolic processes. Aerobic training consists of continuous movements that demand more oxygen consumption and ultimately improve the body's oxygen use. Rapid walking, jogging, running, swimming, bicycling, dancing, and aerobics classes can all be aerobic exercises if they keep the body in moderate to intense motion for a moderately long period of time, with an elevated heart rate representing the body's heightened level of activity.

Most modern-day aerobic exercises are steady state, meaning they're intense enough to raise the heart rate significantly and keep it beating in a very narrow target range for the specified time, which is generally thirty or sixty minutes. Once you hit the desired intensity level, you remain there. For best results, however, aerobic training should be broken up into periods of differing intensities. If you're jogging, for example, you might sprint one block, then jog three blocks at medium intensity, cycling through this four-block, two-speed sequence until you've finished. This is known as interval training, and the intervals are of differing lengths and intensities.

One to Three

The ideal ratio for aerobic interval training is 1:3. This means for every unit of time spent exercising at 80 percent of your maximal heart rate, you spend an additional three units of time exercising at 60 percent of your maximal heart rate. Then you repeat this 1:3 sequence numerous times. For example:

- On the streets, sprint one block, jog three blocks
- On a track, sprint one lap, jog three laps
- On a treadmill or stationary bicycle, go at full intensity for twenty seconds, at moderate intensity for sixty seconds

- In aerobics class, go all out for twenty seconds, then at a moderate pace for sixty seconds

  See "How Hard Is Hard Enough?" below to figure out your maximal heart rate.

The goal is to move fast enough to keep your heart beating rapidly (see below) but to vary the intensity so that the exercise more closely matches the movements our ancient ancestors performed daily. For example, sprinting full speed after an animal, slowing down a bit when they realized they weren't going to succeed in catching it but were still pursuing the herd, exerting more effort as the chase continued up a hill, less as the herd moved down the hill, sprinting all out again as they closed in on an animal, and so on. You can vary the intensity on your own, using a stopwatch or the passage of a certain number of blocks to tell you when to shift or, if you're using a treadmill or similar machine at a gym, setting it to vary the intensity automatically.

For best results, an interval aerobic exercise program should consist of a five-minute warm-up period, followed by moderate to intense interval training involving large and multiple muscle groups lasting about twenty minutes, followed by a cooling-down period of about five minutes at the end.

Your aerobic sessions should utilize cross-training, which means rotating through different aerobic activities. You might, for example, jog or run on the treadmill on Monday, Wednesday, and Friday; swim on Tuesday and Thursday; take an aerobics class on Saturday; and take an intense dance class on Sunday. This will ensure that you use muscles from different parts of your body and will prevent the overuse injuries you might see if you're doing the same activity every day, month after month and year after year.

How Hard Is Hard Enough?

How fast you should go and how much effort you expend during your aerobic sessions depends on the specific activity you're performing and your fitness level. There are two simple ways to calculate this: the maximal heart rate calculation and the talk test.

- *Maximal Heart Rate Calculation*—This formula helps you determine the number of times your heart must beat per minute to indicate that you're exercising hard enough. Start with 220, subtract your age, and then multiply the result by your desired heart rate, which should range between 60 percent and 80 percent of the maximal for your age, depending on the exercise you're doing.

  Here's an example of how to find the 60-percent and 80-percent marks. If you're fifty years old, subtract 50 from 220 to get 170. Multiply 170 by 0.6 (the equivalent of 60 percent) to get 102 beats per minute, then multiply 170 by 0.8 to get 136. So 102 and 136 beats per minute are your lower and upper targets. You can purchase an inexpensive heart monitor to tell you how fast your heart is beating, or you can check it yourself with your finger and a watch. To do so, place the index finger of one hand over the radial artery in the opposite wrist or against the carotid artery next to your larynx ("windpipe"). Push in gently, and you'll feel the pulsations as your heart beats. Count the beats for fifteen seconds, and multiply the number by 4 to get the number of beats per minute.

- *Talk Test*—Start your sprint or other high-intensity interval exercise. Keep increasing the intensity until you cannot talk and exercise at the same time, or until you've exercised for sixty seconds. Now slow down to a mild or moderate level that allows you to talk and exercise at the same time for two minutes. Then start another cycle of a "too intense to talk and exercise at the same time" period followed by a "can talk and exercise" period.

Always Combine Resistance and Aerobic Exercises

No matter how much time you devote to your daily exercise, it's important to stick with the ratio of 2 parts resistance training to 1 part interval aerobic training, always doing the resistance training first. Here's how the ratio works out with differing total exercise time frames.

- 15 minutes total = 10 minutes of resistance training, 5 minutes of aerobic training
- 30 minutes total = 20 minutes of resistance training, 10 minutes of aerobic training
- 45 minutes total = 30 minutes of resistance training, 15 minutes of aerobic training
- 60 minutes total = 40 minutes of resistance training, 20 minutes of aerobic training
- 90 minutes total = 60 minutes of resistance training, 30 minutes of aerobic training
- 120 minutes total = 80 minutes of resistance training, 40 minutes of aerobic training

Core Exercises

Exercising the core of your body—the belly and lower back—increases abdominal and back strength while improving flexibility and balance. This can be done in sets of one to four reps per exercise for each muscle group, with the number of repetitions necessary to create the same burn that you get with the resistance weight training program. To increase the efficiency of your workout and compress its total time, the core exercises can be done during your sixty-second break periods while the upper or lower body muscles are resting. Core exercises include sit-ups, abdominal crunches, leg lifts, and leg scissor crosses.

Time-Intensive Exercise

Two additional steps are required to efficiently and effectively build muscle strength, tone, and contour while simultaneously improving cardiovascular conditioning and cardiovascular health: time-intensive resistance exercises and combined aerobic and resistance training.

1. *Time-Intensive Resistance Exercises*—Performing time-intense exercises means using multiple and large muscle groups simultaneously, with minimal rest periods; for example, lifting light weights over your head while doing deep knee bends. This increases the release of IL-6 and other muscle cytokines, reduces inflammation, increases the helpful lactic acid "burn," enhances postexercise oxygen consumption, builds muscle, optimizes metabolic and hormonal responses, and increases fat metabolism and fat and weight loss.

2. *Combined Aerobic and Resistance Training*—Instead of standing or sitting during your sixty-second between-set rest periods, do another resistance exercise that keeps you breathing hard or some aerobic exercise. For example, on completing an upper body exercise, immediately start doing a lower body exercise or a core exercise that engages large muscle groups and requires "big" action. This busy rest period technique maintains your heart rate and provides more cardiovascular and muscular conditioning. (In a sense, you're using resistance weight training as a modified form of aerobic exercise.) Busy rest periods are similar to supersets in the sense that you are not taking the usual rest break, but you're still resting tired muscles

by exercising others. If you prefer, you can simply run in place, perform jumping jacks, or do another aerobic exercise during the rest period. Other busy rest period exercises include moving your arms in circles, doing hand-grip exercises, and moving around quickly with changes in direction.

Water and ABCT Energy Shake

Hydration before, during, and after the ABCT Exercise Program is vital. Two types of hydration are necessary: plain water and the ABCT Energy Shake. Begin your exercise program well hydrated, drinking about 6 ounces of water mixed with 10 grams of whey protein before you start. (Besides the water-whey, your stomach should be empty.)

Water is essential for optimal cell and muscle function, so you should drink water before, during, and after the exercise session. How much depends on your body size, the ambient temperature, and the length and intensity of your workout. As a rule of thumb, you need 24 to 32 ounces or more during the typical sixty-minute workout and should drink at least 4 ounces of water between each exercise set. If you become thirsty during your workout, you have waited too long to drink water and are already dehydrated.

As for whey, it supplies protein and glutathione precursors, builds muscle, and reduces oxidative stress and inflammation. The ingredients in whey help maximize ATP (adenosine triphosphate) production, improve muscle performance, increase muscle mass, and reduce muscle fatigue. ATP, the fuel for all cells, is synthesized in the mitochondria found inside body cells. Depleting ATP reduces the muscle energy supply, decreases strength, and causes fatigue.

I recommend drinking a combination of water, whey protein, fresh orange juice, carnitine, vitamin C, glutamine, and d-ribose throughout the workout, in addition to the pure water. Consumption of some type of carbohydrates (glucose) during, rather than before, exercise has only a minor impact on fat oxidation when you start exercise in the fasting state. Here is the ABCT Energy Shake I recommend you consume during your workout session.

Into a 24-ounce bottle, put

- 4 to 6 ounces of fresh orange juice diluted with 12 ounces of water
- 30 to 40 grams of whey protein powder
- 10 grams of d-ribose powder
- 2 grams of carnitine tartrate powder
- 1 gram of glutamine powder
- 2 grams of buffered vitamin C

Shake the mixture well. Between each set, drink 4 ounces of water and 2 to 4 ounces of ABCT Energy Shake. Also take 5 grams of branched-chain amino acids (BCAA) in pill form at this time. The BCAA include leucine, isoleucine, and valine.

You can get whey protein, carnitine, glutamine, buffered vitamin C, d-ribose, and BCAA from most quality health food stores, or order it from one of many reputable nutraceutical companies (see the resources section). Be sure to get the highest quality products you can.

Here are the benefits offered by each of the ingredients:

- *Orange juice*—provides carbohydrates in the form of glucose; expending energy while exercising ensures the maintenance of normal blood sugar, despite the glucose in the juice
- *Whey protein*—amino acids and protein for muscles, plus glutathione to reduce excessive oxidative stress and inflammation

- *D-ribose*—immediate ATP production to provide energy to cells and muscles
- *Carnitine*—helps burn fat and provide energy to muscles and the heart by moving long-chain fatty acids into the cells and is an excellent antioxidant
- *Glutamine*—helps build muscle
- *Vitamin C*—helps suppress cortisol
- *BCAA*—increases muscle mass and provides amino acids

Exercise on an Empty Stomach (Except for Water-Whey Mix)

Begin exercising in the morning on an empty stomach, following an eight- to twelve-hour fast. (The exception to the empty-stomach rule is drinking water and the ABCT Energy Shake.)

Many people consume carbohydrates (which contain glucose) before exercise, hoping they will provide energy. However, this actually *decreases* fat burning and weight loss. Exercising on an empty stomach burns more than twice as much fat as does exercising after consuming carbohydrates. It's true that exercising in a fasting state may increase the utilization of muscle protein for energy, but this effect is relatively small and is minimized when you consume whey protein.

Optimal exercise benefits occur when glycogen, the storage form of glucose in muscles and the liver, is depleted. Glycogen depletion triggers the maximal release of IL-6 from muscle, increases muscle growth and fat burning for energy, accelerates fat loss from inside and outside muscle, and heightens weight loss. All of this, in turn, reduces inflammation by increasing the levels of IL-10 while lowering IL-1 and TNF-alpha, increases the production of testosterone and growth hormone, improves insulin resistance, lowers blood sugar and insulin levels, and sets the stage for positive changes in the cardiovascular system, brain, and other organs.

In fact, starting intense ABCT exercise on an empty stomach burns more of the fat stored in and around the muscle fibers, called intramuscular triglycerides. These intramuscular triglycerides are far less responsive to insulin, and their sluggishness slows the breakdown of stored fat. Exercising while fasting maximizes the lowering of insulin levels and the hormonal and cytokine effects of the ABCT Exercise Program. Prolonged low-intensity exercise does not provide these same benefits.

Hormonal Happenings

When you perform ABCT exercises on an empty stomach, after consuming only water-whey:

- *testosterone levels increase*, enhancing muscle growth, mass, tone, and contour; improving insulin sensitivity, which lowers blood sugar and reduces the risk of diabetes and heart disease; elevating the energy level and libido; and slowing aging. Both men and women need testosterone for optimal health.
- *growth hormone levels increase*, improving muscle growth, mass, tone, and contour; improving energy; increasing the sense of well-being; and slowing aging.
- *insulin levels decrease* as a result of the improved insulin sensitivity that develops as lean muscle mass increases. (Lean muscle accounts for about 80 percent of insulin sensitivity or resistance in humans.) This means insulin works better, so the pancreas does not have to make as much. Together, these changes help reduce intramuscular triglycerides and extramuscular fat tissue while reducing the risk of heart disease and inflammation.
- *cortisol levels drop*, improving muscle growth, lowering cholesterol and blood fats, reducing blood sugar, and

decreasing fat in the abdominal area. This abdominal fat is associated with inflammation, diabetes, metabolic syndrome, insulin resistance, high blood pressure, elevated cholesterol, cancer, heart disease, and stroke, so reducing it is key to good health.

Push and Rest

The more intensely you exercise, the more you will benefit. Push hard, to the point of severe muscle burn and fatigue, until you cannot do one more repetition. This is the point of maximal mechanical and metabolic exhaustion, which triggers the hormonal and cytokine responses. After completing the exercise, rest for sixty seconds to allow for optimal recovery of muscle function—but don't wait too long, or you'll lose the benefits.

Especially in the beginning, you will find it difficult to complete the recommended number of repetitions without several three-second rests to allow for partial recovery. Typically, a three-second rest will allow you to do an additional five repetitions before you may have to rest for another three seconds. Eventually, as you become more conditioned, the need for the three-second rests will diminish.

Daily Exercise Utilizing Cross-Training

Exercising daily provides the maximal benefits—and personally, I feel better working out seven days a week. However, it is okay to take a day off if you wish. It is important that you alternate the types of aerobic and resistance training exercises performed every day, so you give your muscle fibers time for repair and recovery and don't injure them with overuse. Doing this also prevents the muscles from becoming accustomed to performing the same exercises each day.

Cross-training will ensure that you alternate your aerobic exercise. You might, for example, rotate between interval running, bicycling, and swimming. Resistance exercises can also be alternated as you focus on upper body exercises one day and lower body exercises the next, with variable core work each day. Or pick two or three muscle groups from the upper body, lower body, and core each day, making sure to select different sets on different days.

Morning Is Best

Exercising in the morning is best, for it occurs after an eight- to twelve-hour fast. This allows for the maximal and optimal production of lactic acid, muscle burn, glycogen depletion, IL-6 release, hormonal balancing, reduction in inflammation, and overall health benefits. Not only is exercise physiologically better in the morning, it's often psychologically better as well. If you wait until the afternoon, there's a good chance you'll find an excuse not to exercise, will be too tired, or will want to eat a snack instead.

Breathe

Proper breathing during exercise ensures an adequate supply of oxygen to the cells, removes carbon dioxide, and prevents lactic acid buildup. Never hold your breath. Breathe in deeply through your nose during the first part of the exercise, and exhale deeply through your mouth during the second part. For example, if you're performing a bench press, breathe out deeply through your mouth as you push the weight up from your chest, then breathe in deeply through your nose as you lower the weight back down.

Rhythmic breathing improves your conditioning, keeps the

pulse and blood pressure lower, and heads off fatigue. It is also very relaxing, increasing the parasympathetic tone that helps with pulse, blood pressure, and heart palpitations.

AFTER THE ABCT EXERCISE SESSION

Once you have completed your ABCT exercise session, enjoy a balanced and nutritious breakfast containing fluids, high-quality protein, complex carbohydrates, omega-3 fatty acids, and monounsaturated fatty acids. Doing so fills your body with macronutrients, micronutrients, minerals, vitamins, and anti-oxidants, which helps increase your muscle mass and improves both your overall muscle performance and cardiovascular conditioning for each subsequent exercise session. Here are some of the after-ABCT breakfast foods I prefer.

- whole-grain cereal with whole milk, raw oats, and wheat germ
- ½ cup of each of the following: fresh blueberries, raspberries, blackberries, and strawberries; you can add banana or other fruits if you wish
- 6 ounces fresh orange juice or another fresh juice, such as pomegranate, grape, or grapefruit—or have an orange, grapefruit, or some grapes
- smoked salmon spiced with lemon juice, capers, hot sauce, and jalapeño peppers
- whole-wheat toast with omega-3 margarine and raw honey
- one or two eggs
- full-fat and low-sugar yogurt with fruit and nuts

Instead of salmon, you might try tuna or other cold-water fish, lean organic meat (buffalo, elk, venison, beef), organic chicken, or organic turkey. Other fruits and fruit juices may be substituted as well. The point is to mix and match high-quality protein, complex and simple carbohydrates, and good fats.

Unlocking the Genetic Power of Exercise

The skeletal muscles are a secretory organ, producing a wide variety of hormones and other substances that "talk to" the rest of the body and influence health. Exercise increases the metabolic capacity of muscle and improves its ability to secrete many of these substances. It does so to such an extent that exercise can change the way genes are expressed, meaning that proper exercise actually turns genes on and off to regulate cell function. Virtually all of the effects of exercise on genes are favorable, improving every aspect of health.

The most obvious change is in the muscles themselves, where modifications in gene expression cause the muscles to become larger and stronger. But that's just the tip of the iceberg; one study found that exercise alters the expression of more than four hundred genes linked to things like:

- upregulation of energy metabolism, decreasing weight and improving energy levels
- improved accumulation of amino acids and proteins
- improved production of red blood cells
- reduced breakdown of protein, keeping cells, muscles, tissues, organs, and skin healthy
- reduced inflammation in arteries and throughout the body
- reduced oxidative stress and free radical damage to cells

The type of exercise done is important in determining these exercise-gene interactions. For example, while aerobic exercise increases mitochondrial biogenesis, converts fast to slow muscle fiber, and improves the ability to metabolize food and nutrients for energy, resistance exercise improves the synthesis of contractile proteins to build muscle and improve muscle strength and contractile force.

In addition, exercise improves the health of the endothelial cells that line all the arteries in the body. It does so by altering the forces on the arterial wall (shear and stress forces), triggering functional and structural changes in the endothelial cells. These changes include increased production of nitric oxide which, in turn, improves mitochondrial biogenesis and thereby decreases inflammation and oxidative stress, opens the arteries, lowers blood pressure, and decreases atherosclerosis.

These and other actions make exercise a genuine "fountain of youth."

GETTING STARTED WITH ABCT: TRAINING SCHEDULES AND DESCRIPTIONS OF THE LIFTS

This section contains different training schedules, ranging from beginner to professional level, to help you get started. Following it are brief descriptions of some ABCT resistance exercises. Always remember these rules:

- Alternate days with the various resistance programs (numbers 1–4) listed below for each of the week's sessions.
- Vary the type of aerobic exercise; for example, running one day, swimming the next, and bicycling the third.
- Do the aerobic exercise *after* the resistance exercises.
- Always do the correct number of sets with each type of ABCT session for the upper body, lower body, core,

flexibility, and balance exercises. For example, if you are doing ABCT 1, do only one set for each exercise. With ABCT 2, do two sets for each exercise, with ABCT 3, do three sets for each exercise, and so on.

- Customize the exercise program depending on your goals and time commitment. If you wish to build more muscle, do ABCT 1, 2, and 5 or ABCT 1, 2, 3, and 5. If your goal is to contour and tone, do ABCT 2, 3, and 4. If you wish to add bulk, contour, and tone, then do ABCT 1–5.

The ABCT Training Schedules

For all ABCT training schedules, specific exercises, such as "chest press," may be cited. General exercises, such as "biceps" allow you to choose from a variety of exercises that work that specific muscle group (chest, back, shoulder, arm, or leg). See pages 177–185 for the lists of exercises for each of the five muscle groups.

Week One: Beginning Session #1, with ABCT 1

1. Resistance training for 10 minutes: Pick the maximum weight you can do for 12 repetitions, and do 1 set for each exercise.
   - 2 upper body exercises: 1 biceps, 1 triceps
   - 2 lower body exercises: squats, lunges
   - 1 core: 25–50 or more sit-ups until maximum burn
2. Aerobic exercise for 5 minutes.

Week One: Beginning Session #2, with ABCT 1

1. Resistance training for 10 minutes: Pick the maximum weight you can do for 12 repetitions, and do 1 set for each exercise.
   - 2 upper body exercises: 1 chest, 1 shoulder
   - 2 lower body exercises: leg press, hamstring press
   - 1 core: abdominal crunches until maximum burn
2. Aerobic exercise for 5 minutes.

Week One: Beginning Session #3, with ABCT 1

1. Resistance training for 10 minutes: Pick the maximum weight you can do for 12 repetitions, and do 1 set for each exercise.
   - 2 upper body exercises: 1 shoulder, 1 forearm
   - 2 lower body exercises: squats with weights, lunges
   - 1 core: leg lifts
2. Aerobic exercise for 5 minutes.

Week One: Beginning Session #4, with ABCT 1

1. Resistance training for 10 minutes: Pick the maximum weight you can do for 12 repetitions, and do 1 set for each exercise.
   - 2 upper body exercises: 1 reverse biceps curl, 1 pull-down back exercise
   - 2 lower body exercises: leg press, hamstring press
   - 1 core: leg scissor crosses
2. Aerobic exercise for 5 minutes.

Week Two: Beginning Session #1, with ABCT 1 and 2

1. Resistance training for 20 minutes: Do 12 repetitions at the maximum weight you can do, then 18 repetitions at 75 percent of the original weight.
   - 3 upper body exercises: 1 chest press, 1 biceps, 1 triceps
   - 2 lower body exercises: squats, lunges
   - 1 core exercise: sit-ups
2. Aerobic exercise for 10 minutes.

Week Two: Beginning Session #2, with ABCT 1 and 2

1. Resistance training for 20 minutes: Do 12 repetitions at the maximum weight you can do, then 18 repetitions at 75 percent of the original weight.
   - 3 upper body exercises: 1 chest press, 1 biceps, 1 shoulder

- 2 lower body exercise: lunges, hamstring leg press
- 1 core exercise: abdominal crunches

2. Aerobic exercise for 10 minutes.

Week Two: Beginning Session #3, with ABCT 1 and 2

1. Resistance training for 20 minutes: Do 12 repetitions at the maximum weight you can do, then 18 repetitions at 75 percent of weight.
   - 3 upper body exercises: 1 upper shoulder and trapezius, 1 biceps with reverse curl, 1 forearm
   - 2 lower body exercises: squat with overhead press, quadriceps leg press
   - 1 core: leg lifts at variable heights

2. Aerobic exercise for 10 minutes.

Week Two: Beginning Session #4, with ABCT 1 and 2

1. Resistance training for 20 minutes: Do 12 repetitions at the maximum weight you can do, then 18 repetitions at 75 percent of weight.
   - 3 upper body exercises: 1 reverse biceps, 1 pull-down back exercise, 1 chest
   - 2 lower body exercises: lunges with weights, squats
   - 1 core: leg scissor crosses

2. Aerobic exercise for 10 minutes.

Week Three: Intermediate Session # 1, with ABCT 1 Through 3

1. Resistance exercise for 30 minutes with ABCT 1–3: Use maximum weight for 12 repetitions, 75-percent weight for 18 repetitions, 50-percent weight for 24 repetitions.
   - 3 upper body exercises: 1 biceps, 1 chest, 1 triceps
   - 3 lower body exercises: squats, lunges, quadriceps leg press
   - 2 core exercises: sit-ups, leg lifts

2. Aerobic exercise for 15 minutes.

Week Three: Intermediate Session #2, with ABCT 1 Through 3

1. Resistance exercise for 30 minutes with ABCT 1–3: Use maximum weight for 12 repetitions, 75-percent weight for 18 repetitions, 50-percent weight for 24 repetitions.
   - 3 upper body exercises: 1 shoulder, 1 reverse biceps curl, 1 pull-down back exercise
   - 3 lower body exercises: squats with weights, lunges, hamstring press
   - 2 core exercises: leg scissor crosses, abdominal crunches
2. Aerobic exercise for 15 minutes.

Week Three: Intermediate Session #3, with ABCT 1 Through 3

1. Resistance exercise for 30 minutes with ABCT 1–3: Use maximum weight for 12 repetitions, 75-percent weight for 18 repetitions, 50-percent weight for 24 repetitions.
   - 3 upper body exercises: 1 forearm, 1 upper shoulder and trapezius, 1 chest
   - 3 lower body exercises: lunges with weights, quadriceps leg press, hamstring press
   - 2 core exercises: leg lifts to chest with floor extension, supine "bicycle" movement with elbows to opposite knees
2. Aerobic exercise for 15 minutes.

Week Three: Intermediate Session #4, with ABCT 1 Through 3

1. Resistance exercise for 30 minutes with ABCT 1–3: Use maximum weight for 12 repetitions, 75-percent weight for 18 repetitions, 50-percent weight for 24 repetitions.
   - 3 upper body exercises: 1 biceps, 1 triceps, 1 forearm
   - 3 lower body exercises: leg quadriceps press, squats, hamstring press
   - 2 core exercises: leg lifts, sit-ups
2. Aerobic exercise for 15 minutes.

Week Four: Advanced Session #1, with ABCT 1 Through 4

1. Resistance exercise for 40 minutes with ABCT 1–4: Use maximum weight for 12 repetitions, 75-percent weight for 18 repetitions, 50-percent weight for 24 repetitions, 25-percent weight for 50 repetitions.
   - 4 upper body exercises: 1 biceps, 1 triceps, 1 shoulder and trapezius, 1 shoulder
   - 3 lower body exercises: leg quadriceps press, leg hamstring press, squats
   - 2 core exercises: sit-ups, leg lifts
2. Aerobic exercise for 20 minutes.

Week Four: Advanced Session #2, with ABCT 1 Through 4

1. Resistance exercise for 40 minutes with ABCT 1–4: Use maximum weight for 12 repetitions, 75-percent weight for 18 repetitions, 50-percent weight for 24 repetitions, 25-percent weight for 50 repetitions.
   - 4 upper body exercises: 1 pull-down back exercise, 1 reverse curl, 1 forearm, 1 chest
   - 3 lower body exercises: lunges, leg quadriceps press, squats
   - 2 core exercises: abdominal crunches, leg scissor crosses
2. Aerobic exercise for 20 minutes.

Week Four: Advanced Session #3, with ABCT 1 Through 4

1. Resistance exercise for 40 minutes with ABCT 1–4: Use maximum weight for 12 repetitions, 75-percent weight for 18 repetitions, 50-percent weight for 24 repetitions, 25-percent weight for 50 repetitions.
   - 4 upper body exercises: 1 biceps front curl with reverse curl, 1 chest, 1 shoulder, 1 triceps
   - 3 lower body exercises: hamstring press, lunges with weights, squats with weights

- 2 core exercises: Lie on back and do leg extensions from chest, supine "bicycle" touching opposite elbow to knee
2. Aerobic exercise for 20 minutes.

Week Four: Advanced Session #4, with ABCT 1 Through 4

1. Resistance exercise for 40 minutes with ABCT 1–4: Use maximum weight for 12 repetitions, 75 percent weight for 18 repetitions, 50 percent weight for 24 repetitions, 25 percent weight for 50 repetitions.
   - 4 upper body exercises: 1 forearm, 1 biceps, 1 upper shoulder trapezius, 1 pull-down back exercise
   - 3 lower body exercises: lunges with weights, squats with weights, quadriceps leg press
   - 2 core exercises: leg lifts, sit-ups
2. Aerobic exercise for 20 minutes.

Week Five and Beyond: Professional Sessions, with ABCT 1 Through 5.

1. Resistance exercise for 60 to 80 minutes with ABCT 1–5: Use maximum weight for 12 repetitions, 75-percent for 18 repetitions, 50-percent weight for 24 repetitions, 25-percent weight for 50 repetitions, maximum weight for an additional 12 repetitions.
   - 5 to 6 upper body exercises with selection from the following: 1 biceps curl, 1 upper shoulder pull-up, 1 triceps, 1 forward with reverse biceps curl, 1 shoulder, 1 forearm/wrist curl/extension, 1 back pull-down exercise, 1 forearm reverse curl, 1 neck exercise
   - 3 to 4 lower body exercises with selection from the following: squats, lunges, quadriceps press, hamstring press

- 2 to 3 core exercises with selection from the following: sit-ups, crunches, leg lifts, leg scissor crosses, leg extensions to chest
2. Aerobic exercise for 30 to 40 minutes.

Chest Exercises

Push-up—Position yourself like a plank, on your hands and toes. The hands should be in alignment with the chest, fingers pointing straight forward, with the hands spaced a little wider than shoulder-width apart. The tummy is tucked in, and the butt muscle is down and straight, in alignment with the back. To work different areas of the muscles, the hands can be moved further apart (more chest) or closer together (more triceps)
Primary area worked: chest
Secondary areas worked: triceps, shoulders

Bench Press—This uses the same movement as a push-up, except you lie on your back and push a weight up instead of raising the body. It can be done with dumbbells, a barbell, or on a machine. It can also be done in an incline or decline position.
Primary area worked: chest
Secondary areas worked: triceps, shoulders

Dip—Best done on a "dipping bar," where the body is suspended and supported only by the arms. In the beginning position, the legs hang down, the body leans slightly forward, and the arms are fully extended. The elbows bend, and the arms lower the body down, then straighten to raise the body back to the starting position.
Primary area worked: chest
Secondary areas worked: triceps, shoulders

Chest Fly—Can be performed using either dumbbells or a fly machine. Lie on your back on a bench with your arms out to the sides holding weights (or gripping the machine bars). Arc your arms up and in from the outstretched position until they are pressed together above the chest, with arms straight out and up. Keep a slight bend in the elbows the entire time. Get a good stretch at the bottom of the movement and a good squeeze at the top.

Primary area worked: chest
Secondary areas worked: front deltoids

Cable Chest Fly—Done on a cable machine, standing, with each hand gripping a handle. Stand with one leg in front of the other, leaning slightly forward, the arms outstretched and back, with elbows slightly bent. The arms are then pulled forward until they are aligned directly in front of the chest.

Primary area worked: chest
Secondary areas worked: front deltoids

Back Exercises

Back Row—Done with dumbbells (one or two), a barbell, or machines. Start by lying facedown on a bench, with your arms hanging down straight and gripping the weights or the machine bars. The goal is to pull weight up toward the body. There are many variations, including close-grip rows performed on a pulley machine and the one-arm version done while leaning over a bench.

Primary areas worked: latissimi, rhomboids, trapezii
Secondary areas worked: biceps, rear deltoid

Pullover—Begin lying faceup on a bench, with your arms extended beyond the head and down, holding the weight. Keeping the arms close together and elbows slightly bent, bring them up over the head in an arcing motion, then lower them back to the starting position. This is usually done with one dumbbell, although there are variations using a barbell, two dumbbells, or a pullover machine.

Primary area worked: latissimi
Secondary areas worked: triceps, chest

Lat Pull-Down—Done using a weight machine. While sitting on the bench, reach up to grasp the bar and pull it down to the top of the upper chest or upper back.

Primary area worked: latissimi
Secondary areas worked: biceps

Dickerson—Done using either a lat pull-down machine or a pulley system. Begin with your arms straight out in front of the body, slightly elevated to forehead level. Grasp the vertical bar. Keeping the arms stiff, elbows slightly bent and shoulder width (or a little wider apart), pull the bar down to just above the hips.

Primary area worked: latissimi
Secondary areas worked: triceps

Pull-Up—This exercise uses body weight only. It is done hanging from a bar and pulling yourself up, or using a machine with a counterbalanced weight bar you stand on for a little help. This is ideal for those not yet strong enough to lift their own body weight.

Primary area worked: latissimi
Secondary areas worked: biceps

Shrug—Standing and holding on to barbells or dumbbells, "shrug" your shoulders up toward your ears to pull the weight up. Arms remain straight down the whole time.

Primary area worked: trapezii
Secondary areas worked: none, or very minor shoulder action

Shoulder Exercises

Shoulder Press—The goal of this exercise is to push a weight up over the head. It can be done with dumbbells or barbells, or using a weight machine. Hand position can be varied. If a barbell or machine is used, the hands can be placed closer or farther apart on the bar. If dumbbells are used, the palms can be facing out (forward) or each other, or changed from one position to the other as the arms are raised.

Primary areas worked: deltoids
Secondary areas worked: triceps

Lateral Raise—Done with dumbbells, one held in each hand, arms hanging down to the sides, with the weights slightly in front of the body. The arms are raised to the side until the elbows reach just above the shoulder level, then are lowered back down. This exercise can be varied by keeping the elbows slightly bent, which makes it a bit harder, or completely bent, which is easier and safer for the shoulder joint.

Primary areas worked: side deltoids
Secondary area worked: trapezii

Front Raise—Similar to the lateral raise, performed with dumbbells or a barbell. Begin with the weight(s) held in the hands, arms straight down in front of the body. The arms are lifted straight out and up in front of the body in an arcing movement, stopping just above shoulder level.

Primary areas worked: front deltoids
Secondary areas worked: trapezii, chest

Rear Fly—Performed with dumbbells, with the body leaning over the legs. It can be done either seated or standing with knees bent and leaning over. Start with weights hanging straight down from the body, level with the abdominal muscles. The weight is then lifted out to the side of the body, keeping a slight bend in the elbows.

   Primary areas worked: rear deltoids
   Secondary areas worked: rhomboids

Upright Row—Done with a barbell or two dumbbells. Begin standing, with the arms hanging down and weights in front of the body, palms facing in toward the body. The weight is lifted up to just below chin level, with the elbows kept high through the motion.

   Primary areas worked: front deltoids
   Secondary area worked: trapezii

Arm Exercises

Biceps Curl—This exercise involves lifting a weight held in the hand by bending the elbow to bring the hands up toward the shoulders. There are many variations, including using dumb-bells, a barbell, or a machine; you can stand or be seated; and the palms may be facing out, in, or rotating through the movement.

   Primary areas worked: biceps
   Secondary areas worked: front deltoids

Triceps Extension—The "reverse" of the biceps curl, with the goal being to straighten a bent arm while holding a weight, then releasing it back into the starting position. If you're using a dumbbell, begin leaning over a bench, supporting yourself with one hand, holding a dumbbell in the other, with the dumb-bell arm pulled back and your elbow bent at a 90-degree angle. Keeping the upper arm stationary, extend the arm straight out so that the dumbbell moves backward and up. This can also be done using a pulley.

Primary areas worked: triceps
Secondary areas worked: shoulder, latissimi

Bench Dip—Similar to the dip but performed using a weight bench to support the upper body with the feet on the ground. Begin with your hands behind you on the side of the bench, palms down and supporting your weight, with your rear end just touching the bench and your legs straight out in front, angling down to the floor so that your heels are resting on the floor. Your fingers should be facing your rear end and the elbows close together. The arms are then bent, lowering the body toward the floor, then straightened so the body is raised.

Primary areas worked: triceps
Secondary areas worked: shoulders, chest

Leg Exercises

Squat—The goal of this exercise is to "sit" then stand up while holding a weight. Starting in a standing position, push the gluteus muscles backwards and lower yourself as if you are going to sit in a chair until you are in a squatting position. Then slowly rise to a standing position. The upper body leans slightly forward, toes are pointed straight out in front, feet are slightly wider than shoulder-width apart. This exercise can be done with a barbell held across the back, or using a squat machine, a Smith machine, a hack squat machine, or a Smith ball on the wall.

Primary areas worked: quadriceps, gluteals, hamstrings
Secondary area worked: back

Leg Press—Similar to a bench press, but it works the legs rather than the chest muscles. Sit or lie down in a leg press machine, with knees bent toward the chest and feet against the weight platform. Push hard with the legs against the platform until the legs straighten but not entirely; the knees should be slightly bent.

Primary areas worked: quadriceps, gluteals, hamstrings
Secondary area worked: back

Leg Extension—Done on a machine while sitting, with the legs down and the ankles pressing up against a padded bar. The legs are lifted with the feet rising up in an arc, pushing the bar up, until the legs are straight out in front of the body.

Primary areas worked: quadriceps
Secondary areas worked: none, or minor hip flexor action

Leg Curl—The "reverse" of the leg extension, performed lying facedown on a bench with the Achilles tendons pressed up into a padded bar or sitting up, legs straight out in front, with the Achilles tendons resting on a padded bar. The legs are flexed, pushing against the bar until the knees are bent, with the heel toward the gluteals.

Primary areas worked: hamstrings
Secondary areas worked: none, or slight lower back action

Calf Raise—The goal is to stand up on tiptoes against resistance. This can be done various ways. The simplest is to stand straight up, feet flat on the ground, holding dumbbells by the sides. Rise up on tiptoes, then descend back to feet flat on the ground.

Primary areas worked: calves
Other benefit: full body stabilization

Lunge—The idea is to "dip" one leg, knee bent, similar to the way a fencer or sword fighter does when lunging with the sword. Begin standing. Keeping the upper body erect, step forward so that one leg is in front of the body and one is behind.

Lower the back knee toward the ground, bending the front leg as well, until the front leg is bent in a perfect 90-degree angle at the knee. The upper body is kept erect. There are many variations of this exercise, including holding the lunge while moving up and down, stepping out and pushing back, and walking. It can be done with dumbbells, barbells, and a machine such as the Smith machine.

Primary areas worked: gluteals, quadriceps, hamstrings
Secondary areas worked: low back, abductors, adductors

Step-up—Holding dumbbells at the sides or a barbell across the back, step up onto a step or low bench (as long as it is very secure and safe) and then back down. It can be done working one leg at a time and then the other, or with alternating legs.

Primary areas worked: gluteals, hamstrings, quadriceps
Secondary areas worked: low back, abductors, and adductors

Abductor and Adductor Toners—Performed with machines, these exercises work the "outside" and "inside" of the thighs. To work the muscles on the outsides of your thighs (abductors), you sit in the machine, legs straight forward and resting on pads attached to weights, then spread them out to the sides. To work the muscles on the insides of your thighs (adductors), you do the reverse, beginning in a seated position, legs straight out in front but spread, then squeeze them together.

Primary areas worked: abductors, adductors
Secondary areas worked: none

Dead Lift—Performed with dumbbells or barbells. Begin in a kneeling position, with the butt pushed back, upper body leaning forward, and the toes pointed straight out. The back is kept in alignment, without rounding. Hands grip the weights, which rest on the floor. Stand up, using only the legs, with the arms and hands acting only as hooking and carrying mechanisms. After reaching the standing position, lower the weight in the same fashion.

Primary areas worked: trapezius, latissimi, erector spinae, gluteals, hamstrings, quadriceps, and psoas

ABCT SUMMARY

- Exercise in the morning on an empty stomach after an eight- to twelve-hour fast.
- Drink 6 ounces of water mixed with 10 grams of whey protein before you start your warm-up or do any exercise.
- Warm up for five minutes with stretching, flexing, and extension exercises of the upper and lower body.
- Start the resistance portion of ABCT based on your present exercise level, time commitment, and desired intensity of workout. Pick ABCT 1, 2, 3, 4, or 5, with varied mixing and matching to accomplish your goals of bulk, contour, and tone. Do the intense exercise until you get the muscle burn. Alternate muscle groups each day for both upper and lower body, and do core exercises.
- Exercise two or three upper body and two or three lower body muscle groups per session, and increase the number of muscle groups exercised with your desired intensity and training time. Do two or three core exercises with some flexibility and balance work as well.
- Ten minutes into the resistance workout, start drinking 2 to 4 ounces of the ABCT Energy Shake at intervals after each exercise set. Drink this first, then drink 4 ounces of water.
- Rest sixty seconds between each repetition unless doing supersets or taking minimal rest periods.
- Take three-second rests as needed to combat muscle fatigue.

- After completing the resistance exercises, start the aerobic program, utilizing cross-training.
- Keep the ratio of resistance training to aerobic exercise at 2:1.
- Exercise daily, but it's okay to take a day off every week if necessary.
- Compress the exercise time and increase training intensity by doing core exercises or other lower intensity exercises during the sixty-second rest periods. Alternatively, you can do the core exercises as part of the resistance exercise session.
- Eat the recommended postexercise breakfast.

Chapter Twelve

New Understandings, New Possibilities

W<small>E'VE LOOKED AT</small> quite a bit of material in this book, much more than can be adequately covered in a single volume. The basic ideas are simple:

- We've been led astray by the myth that the Big Five risk factors for coronary heart disease are the only things we have to worry about—and that if we have any of the five, we must hit the panic button. It's the details of what lies within these risk factors that reveal the true state of heart and vascular health and thus predict the risk of coronary heart disease, as well as point toward the best prevention and treatment strategies.
- Elevated cholesterol and blood pressure, diabetes, obesity, and smoking certainly do not improve your health, but the real concern is whether you have the inflammation, oxidation, and autoimmune dysfunction that trigger endothelial dysfunction and set the stage for coronary heart disease.
- Just testing for the Big Five coronary heart disease risk factors is not adequate, for the simple presence of one of these can lead to misinterpretation of health status and either unnecessary treatment, the wrong treatment, or the

false reassurance that you are in good heart health and therefore need no treatment.

- Research has shown that there are literally hundreds of risk factors and predictors that set in motion the processes that lead to endothelial dysfunction and eventually coronary heart disease.

- Unfortunately, the endothelium has a finite number of ways to respond to an infinite number of insults. They can lead to endothelial dysfunction, which leads to more and more inflammation, oxidative stress, and autoimmune dysfunction. This triggers more endothelial and vascular problems, and the vicious cycle continues.

- Early functional changes eventually result in structural changes in the heart and the arteries. This means early identification of the risk predictors and the resulting changes, followed by aggressive cardiovascular testing and proper treatment, are the best means of effectively combating coronary heart disease. Prevention, *not* intervention, is the key.

I've seen too many patients given prescription medications prematurely, the wrong type of medication or improper doses, the wrong combinations of medications, drugs that interact with one another adversely, drugs that deplete nutrients, and drugs that trigger new symptoms or diseases. I've seen other patients who were given a clean bill of health and soon thereafter had angina, heart failure, a heart attack or stroke, or for related reasons wound up in a hospital or a morgue.

It's time for people to demand the most complete, up-to-date, and scientifically based analyses and treatment of their heart problems available. And the only way to do that is to dig deep, pushing beyond the Big Five to examine many, many more risk factors and predictors. That must be followed by early, aggressive, noninvasive, and if necessary invasive cardiovascular testing. Then, the best integrative medical treatment available must be implemented, with appropriate lifestyle changes, nutrition, nutritional supplements, exercise, weight management, discontinuation of all tobacco products, and the appropriate use of medications. An integrative approach is best, for a wise healer uses every technique that works. It may take some persuading to get your physician to order more tests than are found in the standard cholesterol or heart panel, but it's worth the effort. It's even worth the money to pay for some of these tests yourself at a private laboratory, for knowledge gives you the power to protect your health.

If you have cardiovascular disease or any other problem involving your heart and vascular system, I urge you to speak to your physician about beginning my Integrative Cardiovascular Disease Prevention Program. It's the only one I know of that incorporates the latest information on the proper use of foods and supplements to protect the cardiovascular system, taps into the gene-altering power of exercise, and integrates standard and traditional medicine with complementary medicine. It's the program I use for my patients, and I wouldn't prescribe it for them if I didn't truly believe it was the best.

THE MEDICINE CALLED FAITH

Before closing, I'd like to add a few words on religious commitment and spirituality. More than three hundred studies have shown that religious commitment, spirituality, prayer, and faith are powerful medicines. For reasons we do not fully understand, feeling "linked" to God, a religious community, and/or humanity as a whole resets body chemistry in a positive way. The mechanisms are undoubtedly similar to those seen with exercise and genes, with the good feelings generated by religious commitment, spirituality, prayer, and faith stimulating select genes that, in turn, prompt the body to produce

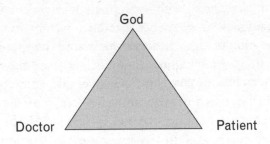

"Dear God, place your anointing,
blessing and healing power and
presence on this medical
treatment and on us."

Figure 3: Healing Trinity Triangle

substances that generate better physical, mental, and emotional health. All in all, religion and faith improve the odds of:

- preventing and treating cardiovascular disease, heart attacks, strokes, elevated blood pressure, cancer, and many other disabling and life-threatening illnesses
- recovering faster, and with fewer complications, following serious illness or an operation
- living longer
- finding peace when faced with terminal illness and death
- warding off or reducing depression, anxiety, and other forms of mental illness
- avoiding or recovering from addictions
- maintaining a happy and fulfilling marriage and family life
- finding meaning and purpose in life

There's no downside to developing the belief that a greater power loves you and has given you tools for bettering your life, as well as facing the problems that come with life.

I'm such a firm believer in the power of faith that I tell my patients about the Healing Trinity, which I believe guides every medical treatment. The Healing Trinity consists of God (or your higher power), the patient, and the doctor, as such.

God gives you both the personal tools to strive for better health and the doctor to assist you, then guides the treatment to its best possible conclusion.

I wish you great health and happiness.

Appendices

In the seven appendices that follow, I take a more detailed look at key coronary heart disease issues. Although I cover the same general ground discussed in the main body of the book, I delve deeper in these sections designed for health professionals and interested laypeople, reviewing some of the relevant science.

Key Cardiovascular Risk Factors

PEOPLE HAVE OFTEN asked me if I could devise a "top-ten" list of cardiovascular disease risk factors/predictors. It's possible to do it on an individual basis, but only after an exhaustive examination that includes a complete history of the patient's symptoms, past medical history, family history, medication and supplement history, and social history, along with assessing the person's use of tobacco and alcohol, caffeine intake, nutritional profile, exercise profile, allergies, surgeries and hospitalizations, complete physical exam results, results from cutting-edge and routine laboratory studies, and results of various new vascular and cardiovascular tests.

However, I can say that certain problems, symptoms, signs, and lab results are very strongly related to coronary heart disease, showing up time and time again in high-risk patients. Some of these are obvious, while others are surprising. Here is my "top-twenty" list:

1. Endothelial dysfunction
2. Increased oxidative stress and/or lack of oxidative defenses
3. Dyslipidemia, taking into account the expanded lipid profiles, particle size, and numbers

4. Increased high-sensitivity C-reactive protein and inflammation
5. Elevated homocysteine
6. Hypertension
7. Age
8. Genetics
9. Calcification seen on heart scans
10. Hormonal deficiencies
11. Diabetes mellitus, hyperglycemia, and increased insulin levels
12. Hypothyroidism, or subclinical disease with increased thyroid-stimulating hormone
13. Increased levels of heavy metals
14. Lack of exercise
15. Lack of sleep
16. Low vitamin K and vitamin D
17. Left ventricular hypertrophy
18. Microalbuminuria and/or kidney disease (microalbuminuria, which exists when small amounts of a protein called albumin leak from the kidney into the urine, has been linked to coronary heart disease, especially in those with diabetes)
19. Obesity
20. Smoking

Appendix II

Homocysteine and Its Effects on Nitric Oxide and LDL Cholesterol

HOMOCYSTEINE IS AN amino acid manufactured by the body and found in the blood. But instead of being incorporated into proteins, as many other amino acids are, homocysteine serves as a messenger, ferrying instructions that directly impact the endothelium and, therefore, the arteries and the entire cardiovascular system. Too much homocysteine alters the environment inside the arteries and sets the stage for arterial disease.

Homocysteine doesn't last for very long, Soon after it's created, it's broken down into two other amino acids, methionine and cysteine, with the help of folic acid and vitamins B_6 and B_{12}. If there are insufficient amounts of these vitamins, the conversion cannot be completed, and blood levels of homocysteine rise, possibly to dangerous levels.

Back in the 1960s, Dr. Kilmer McCully noted that children born with a genetic tendency to produce large amounts of homocysteine had a higher risk of developing serious cases of atherosclerosis and dying young. More than twenty years passed before the links between homocysteine and heart disease, stroke, and blood clots in adults were recognized. Today we understand that hyperhomocysteinemia—elevated blood levels of homocysteine—raises the risk of various diseases. Trouble begins with homocysteine levels as low as 6 mmol/L, with the risk becoming severe when it rises above 12 mmol/L. Problems triggered by hyperhomocysteinemia include:

- endothelial dysfunction
- oxidation of LDL
- increased levels of free radicals
- inhibition of natural antioxidants and free radical quenchers
- increased risk of blood clots
- thickening of artery walls and blockage of the arteries
- increased growth of vascular smooth muscle
- increased levels of cytokines and chemokines that encourage inflammation
- increased activity of HMG-CoA reductase, an enzyme that spurs the production of cholesterol in the body (several cholesterol-lowering medications work by decreasing the activity of HMG-CoA reductase)
- coronary heart disease
- heart attacks
- chronic heart failure (gradual weakening of the heart to the point where it is unable to pump enough blood)
- strokes
- peripheral artery disease (caused by the blockage of the large arteries in the arms or legs)
- vascular dementia (cognitive decline due to poor blood circulation in the brain)
- metabolic syndrome, also known as insulin resistance syndrome—a group of conditions, including type 2 diabetes, obesity, and elevated blood pressure, that raises the risk of heart disease
- kidney disease with proteinuria and kidney failure

Hyperhomocysteinemia sets the stage for these problems by disrupting the healthy biochemical environment inside the arteries. One of the most important ways it does so is by reducing blood levels of nitric oxide (NO).

HYPERHOMOCYSTEINEMIA REDUCES NO

NO is the most powerful vasodilator (artery opener) produced by the body. But rather than acting directly to protect the arteries, it is a messenger molecule that instructs elements in the arteries and blood to perform certain helpful actions. NO protects the endothelium, arteries, and cardiovascular system by blocking several harmful processes, including:

- the "squeezing" of the muscles in the arteries
- the growth of the smooth muscles in the arteries
- the oxidation of LDL cholesterol, which makes it more likely to stick to artery walls
- the clumping together of platelets
- the activity of adhesion molecules that promote inflammation and plaque accumulation
- the adhesion of immune system cells called monocytes to the artery walls, which is an early event in the atherosclerotic process

To put it briefly, NO is antihypertensive, antioxidant, antiinflammatory, and antiatherosclerotic. When homocysteine rises, NO falls, and these protective actions are weakened.

In addition, elevated homocysteine levels can decrease the effectiveness of certain heart medicines, including statins, nitroglycerin, ACE inhibitors, angiotensin receptor blockers, and calcium channel blockers. These medicines, which work by enhancing the action of NO and/or converting to NO in the body, are more effective in the presence of the body's naturally produced NO. When homocysteine suppresses NO levels, there is less of this helpful substance available to work with the heart medicines.

WHAT CAUSES HYPERHOMOCYSTEINEMIA?

A number of factors can contribute to a buildup of homocysteine, such as:

- deficiency of folate, vitamin B_6, vitamin B_{12}, and choline, which are necessary for the conversion of homocysteine into harmless amino acids
- gastric atrophy and malabsorption, which can interfere with the absorption of the above nutrients
- medicines such as diuretics, niacin, metformin, fibrate, resin binders, phenytoin, methotrexate, theophylline, oral contraceptives, sulfasalazine, carbamazepine, and cyclosporine
- coffee and caffeine in any amount
- alcohol (more than one drink per day)
- kidney disease, insufficiency, or failure, which hamper the excretion of homocysteine
- hypothyroidism (low thyroid hormone), which may slow the metabolism of homocysteine
- cirrhosis and chronic liver disease, which may reduce homocysteine metabolism and clearance
- menopause (exactly how is not clear)
- psoriasis, due to increased turnover of skin cells, which increases the levels of breakdown products such as homocysteine
- malignancies, due to overproduction of homocysteine
- old age, due to loss of kidney function
- genetic conditions called methylenetetrahydrofolate reductase (MTHR) mutation and thermolabile reductase

deficiency, which make it difficult for the body to break down homocysteine

CHECKING HOMOCYSTEINE LEVELS

Elevated homocysteine is always a concern. That's why I recommend the level be checked regularly and suggest that a result above 12 mmol/L be cause for a thorough investigation of a person's heart health and cardiovascular risk predictors.

Appendix III

Quenching Inflammation and Controlling High-Sensitivity C-Reactive Protein

O<small>UR NEW UNDERSTANDING</small> of coronary heart disease highlights the importance of inflammation. In this appendix, we'll examine factors that indicate the presence of inflammation, and ways to reduce it.

Factors that cause or indicate the presence of inflammation include:

- increased intake of refined carbohydrates, including sugars, sweets, and trans-fatty acids and saturated fats
- obesity, especially visceral obesity
- smoking
- lack of sleep
- lack of exercise
- high uric acid levels (hyperuricemia)
- chronic periodontal infection, *H. pylori* infection, and others
- chronic infections or chronic autoimmune and inflammatory diseases, such as rheumatoid arthritis, chronic obstructive pulmonary disease, and lupus
- increased levels of heavy metals, such as mercury, lead, arsenic, and cadmium
- elevated serum iron and ferritin

- elevated high-sensitivity C-reactive protein (HS-CRP)
- elevated interleukin-6 (IL-6), interleukin-1 (IL-1 cluster), and interleukin-18 (IL-18)
- elevated tumor necrosis factor alpha (TNF-alpha)
- elevated serum amyloid A
- elevated monocyte chemotactic protein
- elevated soluble intercellular adhesion molecule Type 1
- elevated lipoprotein lipase A2
- elevated vascular cell adhesion molecules

Some of these can be handled directly and without the use of medicines or supplements. For example, you can lower your inflammation burden by reducing your consumption of refined carbohydrates and trans-fatty acids. Avoiding organ meats and certain other foods will help to keep uric acid levels within the safe range in sensitive individuals. You can have your blood and urine levels of mercury, lead, and other heavy metals tested and can take remedial action if they are high. This might be something as simple as cutting back on your sushi and other fish intake or removing dental amalgams that contain mercury to halt the influx of that metal. It may require more complicated therapy to draw metals out of the body.

Taking these steps and others will eventually lower all of the inflammatory markers and mediators, either directly or indirectly. Monitoring will give you a good idea of whether inflammation is being kept in check. One of the most important of these inflammatory markers is high-sensitivity C-reactive protein (HS-CRP).

Heavy Metals and Coronary Heart Disease

We are exposed to heavy metals such as mercury, arsenic, platinum, and copper every day in the air, our workplaces, and even our homes. Some of them find their way into our food and water—think of the mercury in fish. Some enter our bodies through our lungs, and others can even move through our skin into the body. These dangerous substances are everywhere, popping up in aluminum cookware and foil, antiperspirants, herbicides, drinking water, pesticides, fungicides, incinerators, sewage sludge, tobacco, welding fumes, dental amalgams, paints, petroleum products, and more.

Heavy metals can cause a variety of problems, including rapid heart rate, chest pain, depression, muscle spasms, arthritis, allergies, and weakening of the immune system—which can, in turn, open the door to a frightening number of diseases. Here's a brief look at how three of the heavy metals set the stage for disease:

- Iron and ferritin (an iron-containing protein) trigger oxidative damage that can harm the lining of the arteries and increase atherosclerosis. For each 10 µg/L increase in ferritin in the blood, the risk of atherosclerosis in the carotid arteries rises by 3 percent.[1] A recent study of one hundred patients with peripheral artery disease found that reducing iron stores in the body decreased rates of cardiovascular disease and cancer.[2] Ferritin levels were correlated with IL-6 and HS-CRP levels; as ferritin dropped, so did the levels of these inflammatory markers.

- Lead has been linked to atherosclerosis and coronary heart disease, as well as to elevated blood pressure, peripheral artery disease, and cardiomyopathy (enlargement, thickening, and/or stiffness of the heart muscle). Lead damages the arteries by, among other actions, increasing oxidative stress and endothelial damage.

> • Mercury causes oxidative stress and reduces the body's oxidative defenses. It also increases inflammation in the arteries and promotes endothelial dysfunction. Since the body has no way to actively excrete the metal, its level builds up throughout life.

REDUCING HS-CRP

Many things can increase levels of HS-CRP, which is a protein produced by the liver from interleukin-6, interleukin-1B, and tumor necrosis factor alpha. These and other inflammatory markers and substances from arteries, inflamed tissue, fat tissue, infection, bacteria, cancer, and elsewhere go to the liver, where they are processed into HS-CRP. This makes HS-CRP the "master complex" of inflammatory mediators. It's also the best inflammatory mediator for predicting coronary heart disease, vascular disease, and heart attack—and that's been proven by clinical studies.

Although HS-CRP is not itself the cause of inflammation, it acts in many ways to promote inflammation, oxidative stress, and autoimmune dysfunction. This makes it both a predictor of cardiovascular disease and a risk factor that must be kept within the safe range.

Any infection will trigger an increase in HS-CRP, including periodontal disease, *H. pylori*, a sore throat, streptococcal infection, pneumonia, colitis, and sinusitis. Any acute injury that damages tissue will also trigger inflammation and increase HS-CRP. Virtually all of the risk predictors already mentioned will do the same, for the most common final action of these risk predictors is triggering inflammation. If there's no obvious reason for a rising HS-CRP—such as a sore throat or an injury— the increase is probably caused by vascular inflammation.

Regardless of the cause of rising HS-CRP, it is very important to reduce it to normal levels as rapidly as possible to avoid damage to the arteries. For these reasons, HS-CRP should be checked at regular intervals.

Sometimes, the underlying cause of the elevation is a disease that can be identified and treated. For example, a 2010 study published in the journal *Angiology* reported that otherwise healthy adults with chronic periodontal disease had significantly higher levels of HS-CRP and IL-6 compared to a control group that did not have the disease. But when the periodontal disease was treated, the levels of these inflammation markers fell significantly.[3] I've seen elevated HS-CRP in patients with a variety of diseases, including a middle-age man suffering from severe osteoarthritis and obesity whose HS-CRP dropped from 8 to 1 mg/L when both were treated, and a young woman whose HS-CRP fell from an alarming 22 to a very safe level of 2 mg/L when her chronic bronchitis was eliminated with antibiotics. In another patient with *H. pylori* infection, which was causing his stomach ulcers, HS-CRP dropped from 6 to 1.5 mg/L with antibiotic treatment.

In a great many cases, however, the HS-CRP elevation is due to long-term lifestyle and dietary factors. This may sound like bad news, but it's actually good, for it means you can start making helpful changes today. Let's see how some lifestyle changes can reduce HS-CRP and inflammation.

- *Mediterranean-Style Diet*—A 2004 paper published in the *Journal of the American Medical Association* described what happened when 180 men and women suffering from metabolic syndrome were randomly assigned to follow either a Mediterranean-style diet or a prudent diet.[4] The Mediterranean diet is high in vegetables, fruits, whole grains, nuts, and olive oil and low in red meat, refined sugars, and junk food. It also contains healthful monounsaturated and polyunsaturated fats. The volunteers were tested at the beginning of the study and again after they had followed their respective diets for two years. At the later testing, those following the Mediterranean-style diet "had significantly reduced serum concentrations of HS-CRP" compared to those on the prudent diet. Their IL-6, another important marker of inflammation, was also significantly reduced. Fortunately, it doesn't take two years for the HS-CRP level to drop. In fact, you can see changes in the CRP after a single meal: Israeli researchers compared the effects of a "Mediterranean-like meal" with a "Western-like meal" and found that eating the Mediterranean-like meal caused the CRP to fall by 6 percent within two hours.[5] (The Western-type meal did not cause a statistically significant decline in CRP.) A recent study published in the *Journal of Internal Medicine* described what happened when eighty-eight men with slight elevations in cholesterol were randomly assigned to follow a healthy Nordic diet called NORDIET or a standard Western diet.[6] Those on the Nordic diet decreased total, LDL, and HDL cholesterol; insulin; and body weight compared to those on the Western diet.

• *Fruits and Vegetables*—In a 2009 study of the effects of fruits and vegetables on HS-CRP levels, researchers examined the health and habits of 1,060 Portuguese men and women.[7] They found that in normal-weight adults, adding fruits and vegetables to the diet "stabilized" HS-CRP rates, reducing the odds that HS-CRP would rise from the "no risk" to the "moderate risk" category, or from the "moderate risk" to the "high risk" category. Specifically, for every additional 3.5 ounces of fruits and vegetables added to the diet, the risk of HS-CRP rising to a higher level dropped by 30 percent. They also noted that just eating fruits alone reduced HS-CRP, as did just eating vegetables or just consuming more vitamins C and E.

- *Omega-3 Fatty Acids and Fish*—Omega-3 fatty acids, found in cold-water fish, nuts, and other foods, are well known for their anti-inflammatory properties. Numerous studies have shown that there is an inverse relationship between omega-3 consumption and inflammation, with HS-CRP levels falling as omega-3 levels rise. Australian researchers confirmed this in their 2009 study in which they divided 124 healthy adults into three groups based on their HS-CRP levels and measured the omega-3 levels in their blood.[8] Those in the highest HS-CRP group had the lowest levels of omega-3 fatty acids, as well as the lowest levels of the individual omega-3 fatty acids EPA and DHA. In another recent study, Japanese researchers examined the diets and CRP levels of 443 young Japanese women, ages eighteen to twenty-two.[9] The consumption of omega-3 fatty acids was found to be inversely associated with HS-CRP levels: more omega-3s meant lower HS-CRP. Adding omega-3 fatty acids to the regimen of patients taking statin medications for high cholesterol and heart disease further decreased the risk of coronary heart disease and myocardial infarction by 19 percent in the JELIS study in Japan. Cold-water fish such as herring, haddock, Atlantic salmon, and trout are good sources of omega-3 fatty acids, and eating fish has been shown to improve heart health. For example, the DART (Diet and Reinfarction Trial), which involved 2,033 men who had survived a heart attack, found that adding fish to the diet reduced the risk of dying of all causes by 29 percent.[10]
- *Plant Sterols*—Naturally occurring substances found in fruits, vegetables, grains, nuts, seeds, and legumes, plant sterols slow the absorption of cholesterol from food in the small intestines. Instead of moving into the body, the

cholesterol is excreted from the body. Only a relatively small amount of research into sterols' anti-inflammatory effects has been conducted, but the results are intriguing. In one study, sixty volunteers with elevated cholesterol were randomly assigned to take either capsules containing omega-3 fatty acids every day or the same capsules plus 2 grams of plant sterols.[11] Among those taking the omega-3 plus plant sterols capsules, several markers of inflammation dropped, including HS-CRP by 39 percent, interleukin-6 by nearly 11 percent, and tumor necrosis factor alpha by 10 percent.

- *Antioxidants*—Researchers have noted that the levels of antioxidant vitamins in the blood are lower in people who have inflammation, leading to the hypothesis that low levels of all antioxidant substances in the blood—not just antioxidant vitamins—are inversely associated with inflammation. A 2005 paper published in the *British Journal of Nutrition* tested this by examining the relationship between inflammatory markers such as HS-CRP in the blood and the total antioxidant capacity (TAC) of the diet.[12] (TAC includes all the foods and nutrients with antioxidant properties as a whole, rather than the individual elements.) They found that "dietary TAC is inversely and independently correlated with plasma concentrations of HS-CRP," which means that as the antioxidant level of the diet rose, HS-CRP fell. Individual antioxidants such as vitamin C have also proven to be linked to inflammation levels—and taking these substances can help reduce inflammation. For example, when Japanese researchers gave 600 milligrams vitamin C per day for six months to adults with elevated blood pressure, CRP levels dropped.[13] Researchers from the University of California at Berkeley tested the effects of 1,000 milligrams vitamin C per day for two months in healthy nonsmokers.[14] They found that among those with elevated CRP high enough to put them at risk of developing cardiovascular disease, vitamin C reduced CRP levels by an average of 25 percent. Other vitamins, such as A, D, E (tocopherols and tocotrienols), and the B vitamins, the mineral selenium, and micronutrients such as grape seed extract and resveratrol can decrease inflammation.

- *Magnesium*—Researchers from UCLA's School of Public Health looked at data from 3,713 postmenopausal women participating in the Women's Health Initiative Observational Study to determine whether the mineral magnesium played a role in bodywide inflammation and endothelial dysfunction.[15] They found that after adjusting for ethnicity, age, smoking, diet, and other factors, increasing magnesium consumption by 100 milligrams per day led to a 0.23 mg/L drop in HS-CRP, a 0.14 pg/mL fall in IL-6, and reductions in other markers of inflammation. This led them to conclude, "High magnesium intake is associated with lower concentrations of certain markers of systemic inflammation and endothelial dysfunction in postmenopausal women."

- *Aspirin*—Aspirin acts in many ways in the body, including interfering with the production of inflammation-causing substances known as prostaglandins. Back in 1997, a study published in the *New England Journal of Medicine* looked at the actions of aspirin in 543 healthy men.[16] The researchers measured the CRP levels in the volunteers, who were randomly assigned to take either aspirin or a placebo. Among men with the highest quarter of CRP levels, there was a statistically significant 55.7-percent reduction in the risk of suffering a heart attack when they took aspirin. Recently, researchers from New York's Mount Sinai School of Medicine reported that among patients with existing heart disease (acute coronary syndrome), those who most faithfully took aspirin were more likely to have lower CRP levels.[17]

- *Fiber*—Researchers from the Harvard School of Public Health examined the fiber-inflammation link in 902 diabetic women participating in the Nurses' Health Study.[18] They found that the intake of whole grains, bran, and cereal fiber was associated with lower levels of CRP.

- *Weight Loss*—Body mass index (BMI) is a measurement used to gauge whether one is of healthy weight, overweight, or obese. A BMI between 22 and 25 indicates a healthy weight, one between 25 and 30 indicates that a person is overweight, while a figure of 30 or more indicates that a person is obese. Elevated BMI is associated with elevated CRP. This is no surprise, for carrying too much body weight, especially in the central abdominal region, raises the level of inflammation in the body. This was recently demonstrated by Italian researchers, who compared BMI and other weight-related factors to CRP levels in 390 menopausal women.[19] The women were divided into three categories according to their BMI. Those in the highest BMI group were 3.55 times more likely to have elevated HS-CRP than those in the lowest BMI group. When the women were regrouped according to waist circumference and greatest weight increase, those with the largest waist circumference or weight gain were also much more likely to have elevated HS-CRP.

Knowing that the overweight and obese are more likely to have elevated CRP levels raises the question: Does losing weight reduce CRP? The question was addressed in the "Look AHEAD" (Action for Health in Diabetes) study, an ongoing program examining whether lifestyle changes designed to encourage weight loss will reduce the risk of cardiovascular problems and death among overweight or obese adults suffering from diabetes. In the study, 1,759 participants were randomly assigned to receive either counseling designed to encourage weight loss through regular, moderately intense exercise (about three hours per week) and a better diet (which included fewer calories and less saturated fat) or standard care for diabetes. One year later, average HS-CRP levels were reduced by 43.6 percent in the weight loss group, compared to a 16.7 percent reduction in the standard care group.

The link between obesity and inflammation is not just a concern for adults: Swiss researchers working with children ages six to fourteen found that overweight children as young as age six "have elevated concentrations of inflammatory markers."[20]

- *Exercise*—Numerous studies have demonstrated that exercising can reduce HS-CRP levels. For one of these, Greek researchers followed sixty overweight diabetics who were assigned to either a six-month aerobic exercise program or the control group, which did not exercise.[21] Among the exercisers, average HS-CRP fell from 0.48 to 0.29 mg/dL. Their IL-18 dropped from 315 to 204 pg/mL. The researchers noted that aerobic exercise "exerts anti-inflammatory effects" in people with type 2 diabetes, even if they don't lose weight while exercising. Other studies have found that resistance training with weights, rather than aerobic exercise, is the key to reducing HS-CRP. In one such study, resistance exercise caused HS-CRP to fall by 32.8 percent, compared to a 16.1-percent fall in the aerobic exercise group.[22] Since a good exercise program should include both aerobic and resistance exercises, as well as stretching, you'll enjoy the inflammation-lowering actions of both types.

- *Controlling Insulin Resistance*—Carbohydrates from your food cause the blood sugar level to rise when they enter the bloodstream. But the body wants the blood sugar level to remain within a certain range, so it sends insulin into the bloodstream to "corral" the extra sugar and drive it into certain cells to be utilized or stored in the form of fat. In many people the process works well, with the blood levels of insulin rising and then falling back to normal as the additional insulin enters the bloodstream, does its job, then leaves. In many other people, unfortunately, insulin levels remain too high for too long, because they are insulin resistant. They have plenty of insulin, and it enters the bloodstream at the right time, but their cells ignore the order to "open up" and let the blood sugar enter. To get the sugar into the cells, the body has to pump out more and more insulin until there's so much that it "kicks down the doors" and crams the sugar into the cells. The immediate problem is solved—the sugar is safely inside the cells—but the presence of too much insulin in the bloodstream for too long is associated with increased inflammation. Exactly how elevated insulin causes inflammation has not yet been spelled out, and there is debate as to whether insulin resistance causes, or is caused by, inflammation. However, the link between the two is clear, and keeping insulin levels within normal limits makes sense. The best way to do that is to adopt a diet that keeps blood sugar at moderate levels and avoids the spikes caused by eating refined foods, sugary foods, junk foods, and other foods that cause blood sugar to rise too high, too fast. In addition, antioxidants, minerals, and other substances—including chromium, magnesium, alpha-lipoic acid, vitamin C, biotin, EGCG, and fiber—help ensure that insulin works properly and that its levels remain within healthy limits.

- *Reducing Postprandial Inflammation*—*Postprandial* is a fancy way of saying "after eating," so postprandial inflammation refers to the level of inflammation following a meal. The famous McDonald Study showed that eating a fatty meal with refined carbohydrates and saturated and trans fats resulted in significant endothelial dysfunction, high triglycerides, high blood sugar, and high insulin levels, all linked to greater inflammation and more oxidative stress. These abnormalities were reduced if vitamins C and E were taken before the meal. Eating more frequent but smaller meals may help as well.

MORE SUBSTANCES THAT REDUCE INFLAMMATION

In addition to the substances that specifically reduce HS-CRP, many others are known to lower inflammation. They include:

- *Bromelain*—A "protein-slicing" preparation made from pineapple, bromelain is popularly used as to aid digestion. It also has anti-inflammatory properties, as demonstrated in a 2002 study published in *Clinical Immunology,*[23] which found that bromelain alters cell surface molecules required for white blood cell activation and movement, thus dampening the inflammatory response.
- *Cocoa and Dark Chocolate*—Researchers have generated a stream of studies indicating that cocoa and dark chocolate can aid heart health by improving the functioning of the coronary arteries, blood pressure, cholesterol levels, and insulin sensitivity. New research published in the *American Journal of Clinical Nutrition* in 2009 suggests that cocoa may also reduce inflammation.[24] For this study, forty-two men and women at high risk of cardiovascular disease were randomly assigned to receive either 1.4 ounces of unsweetened cocoa powder in skim milk every day or just skim milk for four weeks. Then they switched,

with the cocoa plus milk drinkers receiving only milk and the milk-only drinkers getting cocoa plus milk for another four weeks. While they were drinking the cocoa with milk, the volunteers had less inflammation.

- *Coenzyme Q10 (CoQ10)*—CoQ10 is produced by the body and participates in a number of reactions, including the extraction of energy from food. Animal studies have shown that CoQ10 enhances the anti-inflammatory properties of vitamin E.[25] Laboratory studies show that CoQ10 has independent anti-inflammatory properties, inhibiting proinflammatory substances such as TNF-alpha.[26]

- *Curcumin*—A compound found in turmeric, curcumin reduces proinflammatory substances such as nuclear factor kappa-B and performs other actions that help reduce inflammation while improving cholesterol levels, insulin levels, and other risk predictors.

- *EGCG (Epigallocatechin Gallate)*—EGCG is one of the ingredients in green tea thought to be responsible for many of the drink's health-enhancing properties. For a 2009 study published in the *British Journal of Pharmacology*, Spanish researchers tested the effects of EGCG on monocytes/macrophages, immune system cells that play a role in the inflammation process.[27] They found that EGCG interferes with the ability of monocytes/macrophages to perform certain tasks that aid the inflammation process. A different team of researchers, from Johns Hopkins University School of Medicine, found that EGCG reduces vascular inflammation by increasing the production of nitric oxide.[28]

- *Flavonoids*—There are more than four thousand of these naturally occurring substances found in fruits, vegetables, red wine, tea, soy, and licorice. Flavonoids encourage the arteries to open wide while inhibiting atherosclerosis and reducing the oxidation of LDL, total cholesterol levels, and LDL cholesterol levels. They also have antioxidant and anti-inflammatory properties. A 2007 study published in the *American Journal of Clinical Nutrition* examined the cardiovascular effects of flavonoids by studying data taken from more than 34,000 postmenopausal women participating in the Iowa Women's Health Study.[29] They were divided into five groups according to their dietary flavonoid intake, and the risk of each group suffering certain diseases or dying was analyzed to reveal that a greater dietary intake of flavonoids, as well as a diet including certain foods with high levels of flavonoids, was linked to a lower risk of dying of coronary heart disease and cardiovascular disease, as well as all other causes. Pycnogenol, a flavonoid-containing compound derived from the French maritime pine tree, was found to lower CRP levels in a 2008 study utilizing 156 people suffering from knee osteoarthritis.[30] The flavonoid known as quercetin, which is found in vegetables, fruits, and grains, helps reduce inflammation by inhibiting the proinflammatory leukotrienes and prostaglandins.

- *Ginger*—Known scientifically as *Zingiber officinale*, ginger has been valued for centuries for its anti-inflammatory properties. It acts by slowing the production of proinflammatory prostaglandins and leukotrienes in the body.
- *Grape Seed Extract*—Containing flavonoids, quercetin, and resveratrol, grape seed extract helps increase intracellular levels of the anti-inflammatory glutathione and interferes with the oxidative damage that contributes to chronic inflammation.
- *Hawthorn*—An herb used for various heart and cardiovascular ailments, it has been shown to combat inflammation and oxidation to reduce the risk of coronary heart disease and heart failure, to lower blood pressure and

blood fats, and to reduce irregular heartbeat among people with diabetes.[31]

- *Nettles*—Popularly used to treat allergies, osteoarthritis, and other ailments, some of which have inflammatory components, this herb contains vitamin C, quercetin, and other substances with anti-inflammatory properties.

- *Rosemary*—Known scientifically as *Rosmarinus officinalis*, this herb has been used to treat painful and inflammatory conditions, among other problems. Laboratory and animal studies have confirmed its anti-inflammatory properties, with the carnosol in rosemary being identified as one of its anti-inflammatory components.

- *Lipoic Acid (LA)*—A natural substance synthesized in the body, LA is also found in meat and, in smaller quantities, in vegetables and fruits, although the standard American diet does not provide significant amounts of LA. An antioxidant, LA helps to reduce the oxidative stress that fuels chronic inflammation. For a 2005 study presented in *Circulation*, fifty-eight people with metabolic syndrome were randomly assigned to be treated with either 300 milligrams lipoic acid per day, 150 milligrams of the standard medicine irbesartan, both, or a placebo.[32] Following four weeks of treatment, those taking the lipoic acid, medicine, or both showed a reduction in proinflammatory markers.

Reducing Oxidative Stress

Oxidation is a vital process that occurs in every part of the body, every minute of every day. It only becomes worrisome when it is excessive. The body produces natural antioxidants, such as SOD (superoxide dismutase), catalase, and glutathione peroxidase, and we consume vitamins A, C, D, and E, as well as many other antioxidants, vitamins, and minerals. So in ideal circumstances, there would be a healthful balance of substances encouraging and discouraging oxidation, allowing only the "right" oxidative reactions to take place. Unfortunately, the pro-oxidation factors often get the upper hand, and the results can be disastrous.

The factors related to oxidation include:

- increased dietary intake of refined carbohydrates
- increased dietary intake of trans-fatty acids
- reduced intake of protective and defensive antioxidants, such as vitamins A, C, D, and E
- oxidized HDL
- low levels of PON-1 (paraoxonase-1, a part of the HDL molecule that helps combat atherosclerosis)
- increased levels of heavy metals in blood and tissue, including mercury, lead, and cadmium
- elevated serum iron and ferritin

- too much exercise
- obesity, especially visceral obesity
- smoking
- hypertension
- diabetes, insulin resistance, metabolic syndrome, and hyperglycemia
- dyslipidemia ("bad cholesterol numbers") and abnormal particle number and size
- lack of sleep
- stress, anxiety, and depression
- eating overcooked, browned, or burned food
- radiation exposure
- pollution
- toxins
- insecticides
- certain drugs, such as methamphetamines, amphetamine-like diet pills, and HAART drugs (for HIV infections)
- low oxygen levels that occur with lung disease or time spent at high altitudes
- myeloperoxidase (MPO)

Diet is a major oxidative problem for many of us, directly or indirectly. We eat foods that have undergone oxidation while they were stored and consume oils that are oxidized when cooked at high temperatures (such as frying). We also eat foods that are not yet oxidized but contain substances that either become oxidized or encourage oxidation of other substances once they enter the body. Fortunately, there are many antioxidants in foods and supplements, including the following:

- *Alpha-Lipoic Acid*—A fatty substance made by the body, alpha-lipoic acid is used to convert blood sugar into energy. It is also an antioxidant able to function in both water and fat, which means it can operate in more areas of the body than most antioxidants. It helps reduce oxidized LDL (oxLDL) and recharges vitamin C and other antioxidants that have been "used up" after a single antioxidation battle. Small amounts of alpha-lipoic acid are found in brewer's yeast, rice bran, organ meats, spinach, and some other foods, but the body is the main source of the substance. Unfortunately, the body's ability to produce alpha-lipoic acid falls with age, which is why many people begin to run low in their forties and fifties. When used as a supplement, the preferred form is r-lipoic acid, for this is the form used by the cells' mitochondria.

- *Beta-Carotene*—The plant form of vitamin A, found in carrots, pumpkin, squash, and other orange or yellow-orange foods, as well as in broccoli, spinach, and other dark-green leafy vegetables.
- *Coenzyme Q10 (CoQ10)*—A natural substance produced by the body, CoQ10 assists in many reactions, including the extraction of energy from food. It serves as an antioxidant and reduces oxLDL. In addition, CoQ10 lowers blood pressure; improves heart function; combats coronary heart disease, angina, and chronic heart failure; and much more. CoQ10 levels typically begin to fall at about age thirty, and a great many people have moderately to severely low levels.
- *Curcumin*—A substance found in the spice turmeric, curcumin inhibits the activity of enzymes that encourage inflammation within the body (cyclooxygenase-2 and lipoxygenase). It also reduces oxLDL.
- *Flavonoids*—A large group of compounds with antioxidant and other health-protective effects, flavonoids are found in vegetables, fruits, tea, coffee, wine, and fruit juice. In addition to other actions, they reduce blood pressure.
- *Garlic*—A great antioxidant, garlic decreases oxLDL, reduces inflammation, and lowers blood pressure.

- *Glutathione*—The most abundant antioxidant in the body, glutathione is commonly called "the master antioxidant." A lack of glutathione has been associated with increased free radical and oxidative damage. Glutathione protects against coronary heart disease and heart attack, lowers blood pressure, improves immune function, decreases inflammation, and slows vascular aging and the telomere attrition rate.
- *Green tea*—This tea made from the leaf of the *Camellia sinensis* bush. The active ingredients in green tea, called catechins, reduce oxLDL, improve endothelial function, lower blood glucose levels, and help decrease body fat and inflammation. (See the Antioxidant Highlight section for a brief discussion of green tea's properties.)
- *Lutein*—A member of the carotenoid family, and therefore related to vitamin A and beta-carotene, lutein lowers oxLDL and blood pressure. It's found in egg yolks, dark-green leafy vegetables, and tomatoes, carrots, corn, and other fruits and vegetables that contain red, orange, or yellow pigments. It is not manufactured by the body.
- *Lycopene*—A pigment that imparts a red color to watermelon, tomatoes and other fruits and vegetables, lycopene is a member of the carotenoid family. In addition to being an antioxidant, lycopene lowers blood pressure and improves endothelial dysfunction.
- *Melatonin*—A hormone produced in the brain, melatonin helps regulate sleep. It lowers oxidative stress, inflammation, and blood pressure and improves endothelial function. In addition to being manufactured by the body, melatonin is found in vegetables, fruits, grains, and herbs.
- *N-Acetyl Cysteine*—Derived from the amino acid L-cysteine, it is used as a medicine to protect the heart by reducing lipoprotein(a) and homocysteine levels and for other purposes. It also has antioxidant properties, serves

as a precursor of glutathione, lowers blood pressure, and reduces the uptake of oxLDL by macrophages.

- *Niacin (Vitamin B$_3$)*—A member of the B family of vitamins, niacin is found in chicken, turkey, beef, salmon, peaches, bulgur, and other foods. Niacin lowers oxLDL, LDL, VLDL, Lp(a), and triglycerides; increases the helpful HDL-2 and apolipoprotein A-I; decreases oxidative stress and inflammation; and much more.

- *Resveratrol*—Found in grapes, purple grape juice, red wine, peanuts, and some berries, resveratrol helps protect the arteries, improves endothelial function and arterial elasticity, inhibits blood clots, lowers cholesterol and oxLDL, reduces uptake of oxLDL into macrophages, lowers glucose and blood pressure, and slows aging in animals. It also helps reduce weight and body fat.

- *Selenium*—This mineral is found in poultry, meat, fish, and whole grains, and in smaller amounts in fruits and vegetables. Selenium guards against oxidation by serving as part of the enzyme glutathione peroxidase. It also reduces the risk of coronary heart disease and heart attack.

- *Vitamin C*—An antioxidant found in fresh fruits and vegetables, including guava, papaya, red pepper, cantaloupe, kiwi, and orange, vitamin C recycles vitamin E and glutathione, allowing them to "remain in the fight" longer. It also reduces oxLDL, improves endothelial dysfunction and the ability of the arteries to stretch and contract on demand, improves blood pressure, and decreases advanced glycation end-products.

- *Vitamin E*—Part of a group of related substances, known as the tocopherols and tocotrienols, that have the ability to reduce oxLDL and improve endothelial dysfunction, vitamin E is found in green leafy vegetables, broccoli, brussels sprouts, nuts, seeds, and green beans.

- *Whey Protein*—Found in the liquid that remains after milk has been curdled and strained, whey protein contains peptides the serve as precursors to glutathione. It also lowers blood pressure and improves exercise ability and lean muscle mass.
- *Zinc*—This mineral's most noted antioxidant effects take place in the eye, where it protects against the macular damage that can lead to blindness. Zinc is found in meat, eggs, and seafood, with smaller amounts found in peas, beans, lentils, and whole grains.

ANTIOXIDANT HIGHLIGHT: FRUITS AND VEGETABLES

Fruits and vegetables are excellent sources of antioxidants—and better yet, they provide "antioxidant combos" rather than single antioxidants, which means you're getting multiple antioxidants simultaneously, each with its own approach to quelling oxidation. Several studies have examined the antioxidant effects of fruits and vegetables rather than of the individual antioxidants they contain. One of these studies utilized eighteen healthy adults who ate their normal diets and took fish oil supplements for three weeks, then added five portions of fruits and vegetables daily for the next three weeks, and for the final three weeks consumed their regular diets.[1] While they were eating the extra fruits and vegetables, their blood levels of the antioxidants vitamin C, lutein, beta-cryptoxanthin, alpha-carotene, and beta-carotene increased significantly. Not only did the levels of these antioxidants rise, the susceptibility of LDL to being oxidized into its more dangerous form was reduced. One of my own studies showed that a high dose of a fruit and vegetable extract reduced the progression of coronary heart disease (as measured by the electron-beam tomography calcium score in the coronary arteries) and reduced blood pressure.[2]

ANTIOXIDANT HIGHLIGHT: GREEN TEA

Green tea is a good source of antioxidants, particularly epigallocatechin gallate. For a 2006 study conducted in Portugal, thirty-four volunteers drank eleven cups of water per day for three weeks, then switched to eleven cups of green tea daily for four weeks.[3] Before and after the four weeks devoted to green tea, the researchers measured the total antioxidant status and other indications of oxidative stress in the volunteers' blood. They found that drinking green tea reduced the development of or increase in oxidative stress.

British researchers tested the antioxidant effects of green tea in a group of sixteen volunteers who were randomly assigned to one of two groups.[4] Group 1 consumed a standardized diet for three weeks, then switched to the same diet plus a green tea extract, while Group 2 began with the standardized diet plus green tea extract, then switched to the diet without green tea. While the volunteers were on the diet plus green tea, their blood was better able to combat oxidation, as measured by their plasma antioxidant capacity. But the effect was short-lived, with the increase in antioxidant capacity falling soon after they stopped ingesting the green tea extract. This means that green tea must be ingested regularly to produce ongoing, long-term benefits.

ANTIOXIDANT HIGHLIGHT: MELATONIN

Neither a nutrient nor an herb, melatonin is a hormone manufactured in the brain that helps regulate sleep cycles. Its antioxidant properties have been investigated in a number of studies, including one in which it was given to fifteen elderly volunteers who had type 2 diabetes.[5] Levels of superoxide dismutase activity in the red blood cells and other indicators of oxidative defense were checked in the volunteers, who were given 5 milligrams of melatonin per day. Another set of fifteen healthy seniors served as controls. After thirty days of treatment, there was "an improvement in the antioxidative defense after melatonin supplementation" among the diabetic volunteers.

ANTIOXIDANT HIGHLIGHT: GLUTATHIONE

Glutathione has several duties in the body, including aiding in the synthesis of DNA and strengthening the immune system, but it is best known as an antioxidant that protects cells from the damaging free radical known as hydrogen peroxide, slows the oxidation of fat, and helps other antioxidants do their job. Increasing glutathione levels leads to a reduction in blood pressure and the risk of heart attack and other ailments. In one study, 636 people with suspected coronary heart disease were divided into four groups depending on their levels of red blood cell glutathione.[6] Those in the highest quarter had a 71-percent lower risk of heart attack, compared to those in the lowest quarter.

Unfortunately, glutathione production begins declining early in life, as early as age twenty, leaving many people with a major breach in their antioxidant defenses. Taking the mineral selenium can help patch that hole, for it plays an important role in glutathione peroxidase production and activity. Glutathione levels can be increased by taking special liposomal forms of glutathione orally or by taking several of its precursors, including r-lipoic acid, n-acetyl cysteine (NAC), and whey protein.

A SPECIAL NOTE ON OXIDIZED LDL

In its normal state, LDL is really not "bad" cholesterol. The cardiovascular villains are small/dense type B LDL, the overall number of LDL particles, and the amount of oxidized LDL (oxLDL), or modified LDL. The number of LDL particles drives the risk for coronary heart disease more than any other.

Small and dense LDL is more likely than large and fluffy LDL to be oxidized or modified and then engulfed by the macrophages. It is then used to form the artery-damaging foam cells. The type of fat consumed in the diet determines how susceptible LDL will be to oxidation, as well as its atherogenic properties. The omega-3 fatty acids, which are otherwise highly health enhancing, are the most susceptible to oxidation. Next comes the omega-6 fatty acids, then saturated fatty acids, and finally monounsaturated fatty acids, such as olive oil and olive products. Several nutrients and other supplements specifically guard against LDL oxidation, including niacin, the EGCG in green tea, pantethine, resveratrol, garlic, coenzyme Q10, vitamin E, oleic acid (a monounsaturated fatty acid), polyphenols, and curcumin.

Research has shown that antioxidants inhibit the oxidation of LDL. For example, a study utilizing volunteers in Ireland, Spain, France, and the Netherlands found that "increased consumption of carotenoid-rich fruits and vegetables did increase LDL oxidation resistance," meaning that eating carrots and other fruits and vegetables helps prevent the conversion from neutral LDL to harmful oxLDL.[7] This is not new information: back in 1997, French researchers reported that increasing the intake of fruits and vegetables to the point that they provide 30 milligrams of carotenoids makes LDL less susceptible to conversion to oxLDL after only two weeks.[8]

Antioxidant and Anti-inflammatory Supplements and Other Approaches

W<small>HEN FORMULATING A DIET</small> and supplement program designed to improve the health of the cardiovascular system and the body as a whole, these goals should be kept in mind:

- Control inflammation.
- Control oxidation and improve oxidative defense.
- Control autoimmune dysfunction of the arteries.
- Counteract endothelial dysfunction.
- Counteract vascular dysfunction and improve arterial elasticity and compliance.
- Reduce elevated HS-CRP.
- Reduce levels of inflammatory cytokines such as tumor necrosis factor alpha (TNF-alpha), interleukin-6 (IL-6), interleukin-1B (IL-1B), cytokines, and other inflammatory mediators.
- Reduce levels of intracellular and vascular cell adhesion molecules.
- Increase nitric oxide (NO) production and bioavailability.
- Increase endothelial nitric oxide synthase (eNOS).
- Reduce levels of oxidized LDL (oxLDL) and other modified forms of LDL.

- Decrease the effects of angiotensin II and plasma renin activity (PRA).
- Reduce total cholesterol, LDL, VLDL, triglycerides, and lipoprotein(a) levels.
- Increase HDL, especially the larger and more protective HDL-2B.
- Improve the particle sizes of LDL (the larger type A size is less likely to cause atherosclerosis), VLDL (smaller particle size is safer), HDL (the larger HDL-2B is more protective).
- Decrease total number of LDL particles.
- Decrease intermediate LDL and remnant particles.
- Improve concentration of apolipoprotein A-I and B.
- Reduce risk of blood clot formation.
- Restrain harmful proliferation/growth in vascular and cardiac muscle.
- Keep blood pressure within normal limits day and night.
- Keep blood sugar and insulin levels normal when both fasting and after meals, and be sure that HbA1c is normal.
- Improve the function of the mitochondria (energy producers in the cells).
- Reduce total body fat and visceral fat.
- Stop all tobacco products.
- Exercise regularly.

We don't have a specific supplement or food for each of these goals, and some of them cannot be attained directly; however, they will improve as the diet, supplement, exercise program, and other health-enhancing steps discussed in this book are incorporated.

I can't say which item is most important for you to focus on, for everyone is different. However, I have placed those relating to oxidation, inflammation, and endothelial dysfunction at the top of the list to remind you that while cholesterol and blood pressure are of concern, they are only part of the coronary heart disease equation. Inflammation, oxidation and vascular auto-immune dysfunction are the key steps leading to endothelial dysfunction.

ACHIEVING THE GOALS

The list of foods and supplements that can help reduce inflammation and oxidation, improve endothelial dysfunction, improve the "cholesterol numbers," and otherwise stave off coronary heart disease is lengthy, far too long to permit the discussion of specific diet/supplement regimens centered around each of them individually. Instead, in this appendix, I'll give you some practical approaches for using selected foods and supplements that I've found to be effective and easy to incorporate into a daily regimen. Following that, I'll list the foods and supplements that science says are best suited for tackling specific tasks, such as reducing elevated LDL cholesterol, Lp(a), glucose, blood pressure, and homocysteine, and increasing HDL.

It may seem as if adopting *all* of the foods and supplements mentioned in this appendix would be an overwhelming task—and it would. I tell my patients not to think about doing it all. Instead, pick a few items to start with. For example, just cut back on trans-fatty acids and refined carbohydrates, and start taking one or two supplements that improve endothelial function. When this becomes routine, add a few more heart-protective foods or supplements, or step up your efforts by avoiding saturated fatty acids, sodas, and the refined carbohydrates found in sweets, white bread, white potatoes, white pasta, and white rice. (If it is white, do not eat it.) Keep moving forward, and soon you'll look back in delight at the tremendous distance you've traveled.

Let's begin by looking at sixteen practical approaches.

PRACTICAL APPROACH #1:
CUT BACK ON TRANS-FATTY ACIDS

Fat is not a single thing. There are many kinds of fat found in foods and the human body, each made up of different combinations of fatty acids. You can think of fatty acids as strings of pearls, with each pearl being a carbon atom. The individual carbons are linked, as if holding hands. In addition to holding hands with each other, each carbon may also be holding hands with hydrogen atoms. If the carbons in the string of pearls are holding hands with as many hydrogen atoms as possible, the fatty acid is saturated, or filled up; it can hold no more. If not, it is unsaturated. Some fatty acids, such as the lauric acid found in coconut oil, are naturally saturated, while others, including the omega-3 fatty acids found in fish and other foods, are naturally unsaturated.

The way the links between the carbon atoms are arranged determines whether a fatty acid is a trans-fatty acid or cis-fatty acid. In a cis-fatty acid, the bonds are arranged such that the fat has kinks in it; it literally bends one or more times. In a trans-fatty acid, the way the bonds are laid out causes the fatty acid to be "flat" and straight. This arrangement of bonds makes cis fats pliable while trans fats are stiff, making them more likely to build up in the body.

Most of the fatty acids found naturally in foods are cis-fatty acids. The only natural trans-fatty acids are the conjugated linoleic acid (CLA) found in trace amounts in meat and milk. However, most of us consume a great deal of trans-fatty acids artificially created by food manufacturers who chemically manipulate the fats in foods to give them certain flavor and cooking characteristics, and to make them last longer without spoiling. While that may be good from a culinary and marketing point of view, these unnatural, human-made trans-fatty acids severely damage heart health. Among other harmful things, consumption of trans-fatty acids can:[1]

- increase total cholesterol (up to 8 percent in some studies)
- increase LDL cholesterol (up to 9 percent)
- increase triglycerides and VLDL (up to 9 percent)
- lower protective HDL (2–3 percent)
- increase apolipoprotein B (up to 8 percent)
- increase Lp(a) (up to 4 percent)
- increase trans-fatty acid levels in adipose tissue, leading to more inflammation and oxidative stress; as they accumulate over time in fat tissue, a "reserve" of trans fats is built up and released for a long time, even after you stop consuming them
- change the forms of cholesterol to more unfavorable types by inhibiting various enzymes
- increase insulin resistance, blood sugar levels, and the risk of developing diabetes
- increase the risk of developing a blood clot
- increase the risk of suffering from coronary heart disease and heart attack
- increase the risk of developing irregular heartbeat and suffering sudden death
- increase the risk of developing elevated blood pressure
- increase the likelihood of becoming obese

Where We Get Trans-Fatty Acids

Trans-fatty acids are found in products containing hydrogenated fats, most notably margarine, shortening, and hydrogenated or partially hydrogenated oils. Thus, trans-fatty acids are found in baked goods, doughnuts, cookies, cakes, potato chips, crackers, and other foods made with these kinds of fat.

They are also found in deep-fried foods, French fries, and other foods fried in hydrogenated oils—often the case with fast food.

Avoiding Trans-Fatty Acids

All packaged food products must list their trans fats content on the Nutrition Facts panel, so always check the label. If you see the words "hydrogenated" or "partially hydrogenated," you can be sure the food contains trans-fatty acids and should be avoided. Stay away from shortening, hydrogenated oils, margarine made with hydrogenated oil, and fried foods in general, especially those from fast food chains. If you like margarine, you can find several that are yogurt-based, "light," or contain omega-3 fatty acids and do not contain trans-fatty acids.

PRACTICAL APPROACH #2: EAT MORE SESAME

Rich in fiber, unsaturated fats, and other helpful ingredients, sesame seeds have long been considered a health-enhancing food. Studies back this belief, showing that some components of sesame seeds have antioxidant properties and can reduce LDL cholesterol. A 2006 study involving twenty-six people with elevated cholesterol (greater than 240 mg/dL) found that consuming 50 grams of ground, toasted sesame seeds per day lowered total cholesterol by an average of 5 percent and LDL by 10 percent.[2] Sesame works by inhibiting an enzyme in the liver (HMG-CoA reductase) that makes cholesterol.

One of the substances in sesame, called sesamin, can help reduce the elevated blood pressure that raises the risk of coronary heart disease. A 2006 paper published in the *Journal of Medicinal Food* reported on a study involving forty adults with mildly to moderately elevated blood pressure and diabetes.[3]

For forty-five days the participants used sesame oil for all their cooking needs, and for another forty-five days they used palm or other oils. While they were cooking with sesame oil, their blood pressure and blood glucose levels dropped.

In 2009, Japanese researchers reported on a double-blind, placebo-controlled study involving twenty-five middle-aged people with mild hypertension.[4] Twelve of the volunteers took capsules containing 60 milligrams sesamin per day for four weeks, then took nothing for a second set of four weeks, and took a placebo capsule for the final four weeks. The other thirteen volunteers reversed the process, taking the placebo for four weeks, then nothing for four weeks, and finally the sesamin capsule for four weeks. While the placebo had little effect on blood pressure, the sesamin caused systolic blood pressure to fall by an average of 3.5 mmHg and the diastolic to fall by 1.9 mmHg. These results were clinically relevant, for it only takes a 2 to 3 mmHg drop in blood pressure to reduce the risk of coronary heart disease. Sesame also lowers inflammation by hindering the effects of NFK-B, a part of the cell nucleus that produces inflammatory cytokines and mediators.[5]

Adding Sesame Seeds to Your Diet

Sesame seeds have a mild, nutty flavor that can easily be integrated into lots of dishes. You might sprinkle them on stir-fry dishes, cereal, chopped fruit, steamed vegetables, or spreads used on bread or crackers, to name just a few. You can also try adding a tablespoon or so of the seeds to bread dough or pancake batter or blending them into salad dressing or a smoothie. And there are those who simply eat them with a spoon. (Don't overdo it, however, as ¼ cup of sesame seeds provides more than 200 calories.)

PRACTICAL APPROACH #3:
DRINK GREEN TEA

Green tea, which is made from the leaves of the *Camellia sinensis* plant, is a superior source of a group of naturally occurring flavonoids called catechins. Although there are several major kinds of catechins, the one that appears to have the most health benefits is epigallocatechin gallate, or EGCG for short.

The health-promoting effects of green tea's catechins have been widely studied over the past four decades, revealing that they have anticancer, antibacterial, and antiobesity effects. But perhaps most interesting is their wide-ranging protective effects against heart disease, which include:[6]

- reducing the oxidation of LDL and increasing the enzyme PON-1, which protects lipoproteins from oxidation and inflammation
- improving the lipid profile by lowering harmful LDL cholesterol while raising protective HDL cholesterol
- upregulating the LDL receptor in the liver that helps to excrete LDL into the gut
- decreasing secretion of apolipoprotein B, which means less is available to help LDL deposit cholesterol into artery walls
- reducing the expression of the FA synthase gene, which helps lower fatty acid and fat production
- increasing mitochondrial energy expenditure, which improves energy in all cells, including heart cells

The research supporting green tea's effects on heart health is impressive. In a human study, consuming 224 to 674 milligrams per day of extract containing EGCG, or 60 ounces of green tea per day, reduced LDL cholesterol by 13 percent and lowered the postprandial (after-meal) triglyceride level by 15 to

29 percent. It also reduced the number of dangerous remnant particles. Another study tracked more than 1,500 people in China who did not have high blood pressure over the course of several years. The study found that those who drank ½ to 2-½ cups of green tea or oolong tea per day were 46 percent less likely to develop high blood pressure, while in those who drank more than 2-½ cups per day, the figure rose to 65 percent.

A third study involved 1,900 patients who had experienced a heart attack and were followed for approximately four years. It was found that those who had routinely consumed 2 cups of green tea during the year before the heart attack had a 31 percent decrease in the risk of dying during the four years following the heart attack. Those who drank more than 2 cups per day decreased their risk of death by 39 percent.

Adding Green Tea to Your Diet

Green tea is mild, tasty, and refreshing, so it shouldn't be too hard to incorporate it into your diet. Have a cup first thing in the morning, and sip it often throughout the day. Since it is quite low in caffeine, it probably won't make you jittery or sleepless. The goal is to get 500 milligrams of EGCG twice a day, which is easiest to achieve by taking supplements, and then drinking several cups of green tea throughout the day.

PRACTICAL APPROACH #4: CONSUME OMEGA-3 FATTY ACIDS

Like all other fatty acids, omega-3s are built around carbon atoms, which line up one after another, linked one to the next and "holding hands" with hydrogen atoms. But in omega-3s, the carbon atoms do not hold on to as many hydrogen atoms as they could, which means that these fatty acids are not saturated. They get their name from the fact that the third carbon atom from the end is the first one that has "let go" of a hydrogen atom. (If the first carbon that has let go of a hydrogen atom were *sixth* from the end, it would be called an omega-6 fatty acid.)

Omega-3s first garnered attention when researchers noted that the Inuit rarely suffer from heart disease, despite the fact that they consume very large amounts of fat. But the fat they consume comes from fish and seals, rather than beef or fried foods, and contains great amounts of omega-3 fatty acids. It soon became apparent that omega-3s protected the arteries and the heart.

The heart-healthy effects of omega-3 fatty acids have been tested in numerous research trials, including the following:

- *DART (Diet and Reinfarction Trial)*—This randomized, controlled study of 2,033 men who had suffered heart attacks found that eating fatty fish or taking fish oil supplements could, over the course of two years, lower mortality by 29 percent.
- *GISSI-Prevenzione Trial*—In this large-scale study involving 11,324 people, volunteers were given omega-3 fatty acids, either EPA or DHA, over the course of three and a half years. The omega-3s led to a 20-percent decrease in total mortality, a 30-percent drop in cardiovascular death, and a 45-percent reduction in sudden death.
- *Kuopio Heart Study*—This study found that men with the highest intake of omega-3 fatty acids were 44 percent less likely to suffer from fatal or nonfatal coronary heart disease compared to those with the lowest intake.
- *JELIS (Japan EPA Lipid Intervention Study)*—In this study, 18,645 patients were randomly assigned to take daily doses of either a statin medication or a statin plus 1800 milligrams of the omega-3 fatty acid EPA. After continuing the treatment for an average of 4.6 years,

those taking the statin plus EPA were found to be 19 percent less likely to suffer a major coronary event or non-fatal heart attack than those taking the medicine alone.

• *Meta-Analysis Published in the* Journal of the American Medical Association—A meta-analysis is a "statistical marriage" of existing studies that produces a larger, more robust look at an issue. This one found that low doses of the omega-3 fatty acids EPA and DHA (250 milligrams per day) reduced the risk of fatal coronary heart disease by 36 percent.[7]

These and other studies make it clear that omega-3 fatty acids can reduce the risk of coronary heart disease, heart attack, cardiovascular disease, and stroke. They do this by, among other things:

• reducing inflammation
• improving endothelial dysfunction
• reducing VLDL
• lowering triglycerides
• increasing protective HDL-2
• increasing LDL particle size
• reducing the growth of atherosclerotic plaque and encouraging plaque regression
• reducing coronary artery calcification
• lowering the risk of blood clot formation
• reducing elevated blood pressure
• reducing irregular heartbeats and atrial fibrillation
• improving heart rate variability
• reducing heart rate
• reducing chronic heart failure
• helping the body create stronger fibrous caps to wall off the toxic brew in the artery walls (thicker caps are less likely to rupture and allow the deposits to come in contact

with the blood, causing a blood clot that can trigger a heart attack)

- increasing nitric oxide (NO) and endothelial nitric oxide synthase (eNOS)
- reducing body fat and helping to burn fat
- suppressing ACE activity and lowering angiotensin II levels, thereby reducing inflammation, oxidative stress, blood pressure, and clotting, and slowing the dangerous abnormal growth
- reducing the transforming growth factor-beta inflammation marker
- decreasing microalbuminuria and improving renal function (microalbuminuria, or leakage of a protein from the kidney into the urine, is one of the first abnormalities in the vascular system and kidney that reflects endothelial dysfunction)
- stabilizing cell membranes to make the cells more elastic, responsive, and healthy
- decreasing the occlusion (obstruction) of coronary heart bypass grafts
- reducing stent restenosis (narrowing) following PTCA (a type of angioplasty) and the placement of stents in the coronary arteries
- slowing the telomere attrition rate, which, in turn, reduces the risk of coronary heart disease and heart attack and slows aging

Telomeres, Coronary Heart Disease, Heart Attack, and Aging

Each time a chromosome in DNA replicates itself, a little bit is lost from each end. Rather than lose important genetic information each time—which will eventually kill the cell in which the DNA sits—nature put a protective "cap" at the end of each chromosome. Composed of a string of repetitive DNA, the cap is called a telomere, which is Greek for "the part at the end." With each chromosomal replication, a bit of the telomere is snipped off, but the vital DNA information is protected. (Telomeres also prevent the ends of chromosomes from becoming attached to each other.) Over time, the telomere cap is shaved smaller and smaller until it finally disappears, the chromosome is damaged, and the cell dies. It's felt that this process serves as a sort of "clock" for the cell, telling it when it's time to die.

The original length of your telomeres is determined genetically; some people are blessed with longer "caps" than others. But no matter what their starting length, telomeres naturally become shorter over time and may be subjected to rapid shortening due to inflammation, oxidative stress, nutrient deficits, obesity, and other factors.

Telomere length serves as an indicator of biological age, with longer telomeres suggesting longer life for the DNA, the cell, and the entire person. Your telomere length should correlate with your chronological age or, even better, be longer than average for your age. This would mean your biological age is less than your chronological age and would suggest that you will live longer than average. Since premature biological aging is a risk predictor for coronary heart disease, shortened telomeres also predict heart disease.

New research has identified a link between telomere length and omega-3 fatty acids. A 2010 study published in the *Journal of the American Medical Association* looked at 608 people who had coronary heart disease.[8] The length of telomeres in their white blood cells and their levels of the omega-3 fatty acids EPA and DHA were measured at the beginning of the study. Five years later, telomere length was checked again. There was an inverse relationship between telomere length and omega-3 fatty acid levels, meaning that those with the highest omega-3 levels suffered less telomere shortening than did those with the lowest omega-3 levels. The results of this study supported those of a 2007 study published in the prestigious journal *Lancet*, which found that among middle-age, high-risk men, telomere length in white blood cells "is a predictor of future coronary heart disease."[9]

Increasing the intake of omega-3 fatty acids is not the only way to slow the shortening of telomeres. Other approaches include lowering oxidative stress while increasing oxidative defenses; reducing inflammation, blood pressure, lipids, oxLDL, glucose, and homocysteine; slimming down to your ideal weight, eating so as to get optimal nutrition and significantly restricting caloric intake; getting plenty of sleep; giving up smoking; increasing nitric oxide, vitamin D, and estrogen levels; and exercising more. Various supplements, including resveratrol, vitamin K_2 MK7, glutathione, and other antioxidants, are also helpful. Finally, certain medications can slow telomere attrition rate. These include the angiotensin converting enzyme inhibitors and angiotensin receptor blockers used to treat hypertension and heart disease, the statins prescribed to treat high cholesterol, the diabetes medicine metformin, hormone replacement therapy, and aspirin.

Adding Omega-3 Fatty Acids to Your Diet

Omega-3 fatty acids are found primarily in cold-water fatty fish such as salmon, mackerel, herring, and tuna. Be aware that fish raised on fish farms are lower in omega-3s than wild-caught fish, due to the content of their diets. Other sources of omega-3s include fish oil, krill, and algae.

Precursors of omega-3s are flax, flaxseed, and flax oil, but these are less efficient foods for getting omega-3s into your system, as the body has to convert them. Not only is the conversion rate to DHA and EPA less than 5 percent, but these precursors may go into the inflammatory omega-6 pathway instead, increasing inflammation and coronary heart disease risk in some patients. They are not recommended.

The goal is a daily intake of 3 to 4 grams of EPA and DHA combined in a ratio of 3 parts EPA to 2 parts DHA. A 3-ounce serving of Pacific herring or Pacific oysters provides about 1.8 grams of EPA/DHA in the recommended ratio, while a 3-ounce serving of Chinook salmon provides about 1.5 grams. Supplements of fish oil or krill oil can make up the shortfall. It's also recommended that the 3 to 4 grams of EPA/DHA be balanced with 1.5 to 2 grams (about 50 percent of that total) gamma-linolenic acid (GLA) and 100 to 200 international units gamma-/delta-vitamin E daily.

PRACTICAL APPROACH #5: EAT MORE FIBER

Fiber, also called dietary fiber or roughage, consists of the parts of plant foods we cannot digest. Some kinds of fiber are soluble, which means they become a gelatinous substance when fermented by bacteria in the digestive tract. Others are insoluble or inert; they absorb water, are not fermented, and pass through the digestive system intact. As a general rule, soluble fiber helps "mop up" excess cholesterol and escort it out of the body, while insoluble fiber improves bowel function by bulking up the stool. Plant foods typically contain both types of fiber in varying proportions. Although fiber itself has no nutritional value—it simply passes through the gastrointestinal tract—it can change the way certain other substances behave and thus exert a major impact on health.

Consuming ample amounts of soluble fiber reduces the risk of suffering from coronary heart disease as well as cardiovascular disease. Specifically, soluble fiber reduces blood glucose and insulin levels, total cholesterol, LDL cholesterol, and triglycerides. The average LDL reduction due to soluble fiber seen in randomized, controlled trials is 10 percent.

Insoluble fiber has been associated with a decrease in cardiovascular disease, a slower progression of existing disease, and a modest reduction in the risk of heart attack. Insoluble fiber also increases the feeling of fullness, reducing consumption of calories and lowering the risk of obesity.

Adding Fiber to Your Diet

The goal is to consume 30 to 50 grams of total fiber per day from food, not supplements. At least 10 grams should be from soluble fiber. Insoluble fiber is found in whole grains, legumes, fresh vegetables, and fruits (eat with the skin on, if possible). Good sources of soluble fiber include oats, legumes, fruits, barley, and psyllium seed.

PRACTICAL APPROACH #6: EAT GARLIC

Thousands of years ago, the Chinese prized garlic it for its ability to thin the blood, and the ancient Greeks used it to enhance athletic performance at the Olympic Games. In recent times, thirteen different placebo-controlled studies involving 781 patients receiving 600 to 900 milligrams per day of a standardized garlic extract found that garlic reduced total cholesterol by an average of 16 percent. The results were not consistent, however, and some studies showed no benefit at all. This disagreement between studies is a common problem in medical research, often caused by the fact that different studies use different groups of subjects, use different brands of extract, run for different lengths of time, and include other variations that lead to contradictory results. However, there is enough evidence to suggest that garlic can protect against coronary heart disease by reducing LDL oxidation and by lowering total cholesterol in some people.

Adding Garlic to Your Diet

There are lots of ways to add more garlic to your diet. Add chopped or minced garlic to soups, stews, stir-fry dishes, salads, and mashed potatoes. Sauté your vegetables in water, broth or a little oil plus chopped garlic. Use garlic-based marinades for seafood, poultry, and meat. Put an entire bulb of garlic into a pot of broth while you're cooking it, then strain the garlic pieces out. You'll increase your garlic quotient and enjoy a tastier broth at the same time.

PRACTICAL APPROACH #7: CONSIDER TAKING SUPPLEMENTAL NIACIN

Niacin, a member of B family of vitamins that is also known as vitamin B_3, has been used to promote heart health since the mid-1900s. Although it has been pushed aside by cholesterol-lowering medications, niacin's ability to lower cholesterol is widely recognized. Studies have shown that daily doses of 1 to 4 grams of niacin per day can lead to:

- a decrease in total cholesterol of 20 to 25 percent
- a decrease in LDL of 10 to 25 percent, particularly the more harmful small, dense LDL
- a decrease in triglycerides of 20 to 25 percent
- an increase in HDL of 15 to 35 percent, especially the more heart protective HDL-2

Niacin's properties go beyond pushing the "cholesterol numbers" in a heart-healthy direction. It also:

- functions as a potent antioxidant
- lowers small dense LDL, shifts the harmful LDL-B pattern to the better LDL-A pattern, and reduces the LDL particle number
- inhibits LDL oxidation
- reduces Lp(a)
- lowers apolipoprotein B
- lowers triglycerides
- increases helpful HDL-2B
- inhibits platelet function, thereby helping to prevent unwanted blood clots
- inhibits cytokines, cell adhesion molecules, and other inflammation markers

The results of a randomized, placebo-controlled trial called the Coronary Drug Project that involved 3,908 men showed that niacin reduced the incidence of nonfatal heart attacks by 26 percent and cerebrovascular events by 24 percent over the course of six years. After fifteen years of follow-up, total mortality was 11-percent lower in the niacin group than in the placebo group.[10]

Taking Niacin

Niacin should always be taken with food. Begin with 100 milligrams day, slowly increasing the dose by 100 milligrams per week until a good response occurs. It is helpful to take a baby aspirin every day prior to the niacin, to help reduce flushing. Eating an apple or applesauce also helps reduce flushing. Do not drink alcohol at the time you take niacin.

Niacin's potential side effects include flushing, rash, elevated blood sugar, elevated levels of uric acid, and an increased risk of developing gout, hepatitis, rash, gastritis, peptic ulcer disease, bruising, and irregular heartbeat. Most of these are dose-related side effects, so beginning with a small dose and monitoring your reaction carefully as you increase it will help you catch any side effects early on and counter them by reducing the dose. Also remember that the nonflush niacin supplements sold over the counter do not work. They are composed of a different compound called IHN and, when compared to flush niacin (vitamin B_3) in clinical studies, are ineffective.

PRACTICAL APPROACH #8: CONSIDER TAKING SUPPLEMENTAL TOCOTRIENOLS

Vitamin E is not a single substance. Instead, it is a group of eight different substances with similar actions in the body. The eight substances are divided into two groups, called tocotrienols and tocopherols. There are four of each—alpha-tocotrienol, beta-tocotrienol, delta-tocotrienol, and gamma-tocotrienol in the former group, and alpha-tocopherol, beta-tocopherol, delta-tocopherol, and gamma-tocopherol in the latter. When a food or supplement is said to contain vitamin E, it actually contains one or more of these eight forms. Eating a variety of foods will ensure that you get ample amounts of these various forms. Supplements, however, often only contain one or a few of the eight forms, which can render the supplement ineffective.

Research into the properties of the various forms of vitamin E have made it clear that it's the tocotrienols that are helpful in protecting the heart. Epidemiologic studies, which look at the health and habits of large groups of people, have shown that a diet rich in foods that contain high levels of tocotrienols, such as cereal grains, vegetables, and fruits, reduces the risk of suffering from cardiovascular disease.

Studies have shown that the tocotrienols can improve the

cholesterol profile. A 2002 study found that 100 milligrams per day of a tocotrienol-rich supplement called TRF25 reduces:[11]

- total cholesterol as much as 20 percent
- LDL as much as 25 percent
- apolipoprotein B as much as 14 percent
- triglycerides as much as 12 percent

Laboratory research indicates that the tocotrienols also have antioxidant properties.[12]

Taking Tocotrienols

I recommend a supplement containing 100 milligrams of gamma-/delta-tocotrienols. Take it with your evening meal, and make sure that twelve hours have passed since taking any other form of vitamin E, especially alpha-tocopherol. If you take alpha-tocopherol, it should amount to less than 20 percent of the total amount of tocopherols you consume via supplements each day. This allows better absorption of the tocotrienols and distribution to the tissues.

PRACTICAL APPROACH #9:
CONSIDER TAKING SUPPLEMENTAL
PANTETHINE

Pantethine is a derivative of pantothenic acid (vitamin B_5). This doesn't mean it's unnatural, as all of the vitamins undergo various transformations within the body, and the various derivatives of vitamins have different properties and are used in different ways. Pantethine's properties include reducing cholesterol and otherwise protecting the heart. Twenty-eight different studies involving 646 people have shown that it:[13]

- lowers total cholesterol 15 percent
- lowers LDL 20 percent
- lowers apolipoprotein B up to 27.6 percent
- increases HDL 8 percent
- increases apolipoprotein A-I
- lowers triglycerides 33 percent

In addition, panthetine

- reduces the deposition of fats and the development of fatty streaks in the aorta and coronary arteries
- reduces intimal (arterial wall) thickening in the aorta and coronary arteries
- reduces LDL oxidation

Taking Pantethine

Take 300 milligrams of pantethine three times a day, or 450 milligrams twice a day. Peak effects usually occur after four months of supplementation, but it may take six to nine months to see them.

PRACTICAL APPROACH #10: CONSIDER TAKING SUPPLEMENTAL CHROMIUM IF YOU ARE DEFICIENT

Chromium is a trace mineral, meaning that humans require only small amounts for good health. It's measured in micrograms (mcg) rather than milligrams or grams, for the quantity in the body is relatively tiny. However, even in small amounts, chromium performs important tasks, helping to:

- reduce total cholesterol
- increase HDL

- keep blood sugar levels under control and reduce insulin resistance, thereby protecting against diabetes-related damage to the arteries
- reduce fasting blood glucose

Taking Chromium

Take supplements only if you are deficient in the mineral. Chromium is found in meat, cheese, beer, whole grains, and other foods. I recommend a daily intake of 200 to 800 micrograms.

PRACTICAL APPROACH #11: CONSIDER TAKING SUPPLEMENTAL COENZYME Q10

Coenzyme Q10 (CoQ10) is naturally produced by the body and is necessary for proper cell function. It's found in concentrated amounts in tissues and organs that need a lot of energy, like the heart. CoQ10 levels tend to fall with age and are low in some people suffering from chronic heart disease, cancer, diabetes, and other long-term illnesses.

Although CoQ10 does not improve total cholesterol, LDL, or HDL levels, it has antioxidant properties, protects LDL from oxidation, reduces Lp(a) levels, and improves endothelial dysfunction. Unfortunately, taking a statin medication such as Lipitor (atorvastatin), as millions of people do, can cause the body to run short of CoQ10—an ironic situation, for the medicines designed to help the heart also harm it by depriving it of a natural protector. For this reason, everyone taking a statin medicine should get their CoQ10 levels measured and, if they are low, consider taking CoQ10 supplements.

Even for those who do not take statin medications, CoQ10 supplements can be a worthwhile addition to any program designed to reduce inflammation and oxidation, control cholesterol, and otherwise build good health.

Taking CoQ10

Either use a highly absorbable form labeled "nano" or "combined with liposome or fat delivery system" or take CoQ10 with small amounts of fatty foods to increase absorption. One hundred to 200 milligrams per day is usually enough, but higher doses are indicated in certain heart conditions or with severe depletion. CoQ10 is safe even in very high doses.

PRACTICAL APPROACH #12: CONSIDER TAKING SUPPLEMENTAL CHINESE RED YEAST RICE

Chinese red yeast rice is rice fermented by the red yeast known as *Monascus purpureus.* The resulting product has properties similar to those of the statin medications used to control cholesterol levels. Numerous studies have shown that Chinese red yeast rice can

- lower LDL 22 to 32 percent
- lower total cholesterol 16 to 31 percent
- lower triglycerides by up to 36 percent
- raise HDL by up to 20 percent

Chinese red yeast rice does this by interfering with the synthesis of cholesterol in the body.

Taking Chinese Red Yeast Rice

Take 2,400 to 4,800 milligrams of Chinese red yeast rice at night with food. Do not buy it over the counter or on the Internet, for Chinese red yeast rice must be pure and free from contaminants. Only use a supplement from a highly reputable source such as Biotics Research of Texas.

PRACTICAL APPROACH #13: CONSIDER TAKING SUPPLEMENTAL PLANT STEROLS

Plant sterols are a group of phytochemicals called steroid alcohols that occur naturally in plant foods such as vegetables, fruits, and other foods grown in the ground, but not in foods of animal origin. Because they are molecularly similar to cholesterol, they can "elbow aside" cholesterol found in the digestive tract and prevent it from being absorbed into the body.

Several studies[14] have looked at the cholesterol-lowering effects of plant sterols, demonstrating that they can lower total cholesterol by 8 percent and lower LDL cholesterol by 10 percent while reducing the progression of atherosclerosis and intima media thickness and speeding regression of the plaques that threaten to trigger heart attacks and strokes.

Taking Plant Sterols

Take 2 grams per day. It is very safe and effective.

PRACTICAL APPROACH #14: CONSIDER TAKING SUPPLEMENTAL POLYPHENOLS AND RESVERATROL

Polyphenols are naturally occurring compounds with powerful antioxidant properties that are found in green tea, apples, olive oil, walnuts, pomegranates, cocoa, and other foods of plant origin. The polyphenols can be further classified into flavonoids, lignins, phenolic acids, and stilbenes.

One of the more famous polyphenols is a stilbene called resveratrol that is found in the skin of grapes, purple grape juice, red wine, peanuts, and some berries. It reduces cholesterol and helps "thin" the blood, thereby preventing unnecessary and potentially harmful blood clots.

Research into polyphenols in general and resveratrol in particular has shown that they:

- reduce inflammation and increase levels of the anti-inflammatory nitric oxide (NO)
- have antioxidant properties
- reduce LDL oxidation
- improve endothelial dysfunction
- increase the activity of PON-1, a liver enzyme that helps prevent the oxidation of HDL
- improve the ability of the blood vessels to relax and widen when appropriate
- reduce atherosclerosis (in animals)
- reduce total cholesterol, LDL, and triglycerides
- protect telomeres and slow the aging of the arteries
- help reduce body fat
- lower glucose and improve insulin resistance

Taking Resveratrol and Polyphenols

Only take resveratrol in the trans-resveratrol form, 250 to 350 milligrams per day, purchased from a highly reputable source such as Biotics Research. Do not take more than this, for clinical studies suggest that humans have the best response to this dose.

PRACTICAL APPROACH #15: CONSIDER TAKING SUPPLEMENTAL VITAMIN C

A water-soluble vitamin found in citrus fruit, guava, red and green peppers, strawberries, and other foods, vitamin C is a powerful antioxidant that "recycles" vitamin E and improves endothelial dysfunction. Levels of the vitamin are inversely related to blood pressure, with the diastolic and systolic blood pressure falling as vitamin C intake rises. Studies of large populations show that the risk of coronary heart disease decreases as vitamin C consumption increases. Vitamin C's specific actions include:

- combating oxidation
- lowering the levels of total cholesterol, LDL cholesterol, and triglycerides while increasing HDL
- improving the elasticity and performance of the large artery called the aorta
- reducing the formation of a blood clot (thrombosis)

Taking Vitamin C

Take 250 to 500 milligrams of vitamin C daily. Higher doses are safe but may cause diarrhea.

PRACTICAL APPROACH #16: CONSIDER TAKING SUPPLEMENTAL CURCUMIN

Found in the spice turmeric (commonly used in East Indian curries), curcumin has antioxidant, anti-inflammatory, and cholesterol-lowering properties. In a study of ten healthy people who were given 500 milligrams of curcumin per day for ten days, the levels of oxidizing agents called serum lipid peroxides fell by 33 percent, total cholesterol dropped by 11.6 percent, and HDL rose by 29 percent.

Taking Curcumin

Take 500 milligrams per day, but be sure to use high-quality curcumin to get all the benefits. Curcumin's side effects include nausea and diarrhea, and it may increase bleeding time in people who are taking anticoagulant medicines or supplements.

Expanded Supplement Regimens
for Specific Problems Related to CAD

IN THE MAIN TEXT of this book, I outlined supplement programs designed to help reduce inflammation, oxidation, dyslipidemia, disturbances in blood pressure and flow, and problems with blood glucose and insulin. In this section, I offer lengthier, targeted interventions for certain specific predictors of coronary heart disease. The items listed in each Attack Plan are backed by solid scientific evidence and the best clinical data available.

ATTACK PLAN #1: TO LOWER THE RISK
OF SUFFERING A HEART ATTACK

- Acetyl l-carnitine (ALCAR)—500 milligrams twice per day
- Alpha-lipoic acid (ALA)—100 to 200 milligrams per day, use only the isomer called r-lipoic acid
- B complex with natural folates—400 micrograms per day
- Coenzyme Q10—100 milligrams per day
- EGCG (epigallocatechin gallate)—500 milligrams twice per day
- Fiber—50 grams of mixed fiber per day
- Lutein—5 milligrams per day

- Lycopene—20 milligrams per day
- Magnesium chelates—500 milligrams twice per day
- Mediterranean diet with lots of olive oil and olives to provide monounsaturated fatty acids
- Niacin—500 to 1,000 milligrams per day
- Omega-3 fatty acids—3 to 5 grams per day
- Trans-resveratrol—250 to 300 milligrams per day
- Vitamin C—250 milligrams twice per day
- Vitamin D—increase the blood level to 50–60 ng/mL
- Vitamin K_2 MK7—100 to 150 micrograms per day

Vitamin K comes in different forms, as do many other vitamins. The K_2 form has been shown to protect the heart and cardiovascular system, while the K_1 form has no such protective effects. In the Rotterdam Study, vitamin K_2 reduced the risk of coronary heart disease 57 percent in those consuming the largest amount of the vitamin, compared to those taking the lowest amount.[1] It also reduced dangerous calcification in the aorta by 52 percent and the overall risk of dying by 26 percent. The most heart-protective form of the vitamin is known as vitamin K_2 MK7.

ATTACK PLAN #2: TO INHIBIT
LDL OXIDATION

- CoQ10 (coenzyme Q10)—100 to 200 milligrams per day
- Curcumin (turmeric)—1 to 2 tablespoons per day on food or in standardized supplement form
- EGCG—500 milligrams twice per day
- Garlic—1 to 2 cloves per day
- Niacin—500 to 1,000 milligrams per day
- Oleic acid (a monounsaturated fatty acid, or MUFA)— 5 tablespoons of extra virgin olive oil on salads and food per day

- Pantethine—450 milligrams twice per day
- Polyphenols—a wide variety of fruits and vegetables, red wine, grapes, and raisins
- Trans-resveratrol—250 to 350 milligrams per day
- Vitamin E—100 milligrams of gamma-/delta-tocotrienols per day

ATTACK PLAN #3: TO CONVERT DENSE TYPE B LDL TO LARGE TYPE A LDL

- Niacin—500 to 1,000 milligrams per day
- Omega-3 fatty acids—3 to 5 grams per day
- Plant sterols—2 grams per day
- Reduce blood triglycerides to below 75 percent
- Reduce intake of refined carbohydrates
- Water-soluble fiber—50 grams per day

ATTACK PLAN #4: TO LOWER LP(A)

- Alcohol (red wine)—about 6 ounces per day
- Aspirin—81 milligrams per day
- CoQ10—100 to 200 milligrams per day
- Estrogen bioidentical hormone replacement
- Exercise (see chapter eleven for a discussion of the optimal exercise program)
- L-carnitine—2,000 milligrams twice per day
- N-acetyl cysteine—500 to 1,000 milligrams twice per day
- Niacin—500 to 1,000 milligrams per day
- Omega-3 fatty acids—3 to 5 grams per day
- Vitamin C—3 grams per day or more
- Vitamin E—100 milligrams of gamma-/delta-tocotrienols per day

ATTACK PLAN #5: TO INCREASE HDL-2 AND/OR CONVERT HDL-3 TO HDL-2

- Alcohol (red wine)—about 6 ounces per day
- Exercise (see chapter eleven for a discussion of the optimal exercise program)
- Niacin—500 to 1,000 milligrams per day
- Omega-3 fatty acids—3 to 5 grams per day
- Pantethine—450 milligrams twice per day
- Reduce intake of trans-fatty acids and saturated fatty acids
- Slim down to healthy weight
- Stop smoking

ATTACK PLAN #6: TO REDUCE CHOLESTEROL ABSORPTION IN INTESTINES

- EGCG—500 milligrams twice per day
- Fiber—50 grams of mixed fiber per day
- Plant sterols—2 grams per day
- Sesame—40 grams per day

ATTACK PLAN #7: TO LOWER TOTAL CHOLESTEROL AND LDL

- Niacin—500 to 1,000 milligrams per day
- Omega-3 fatty acids—3 to 5 grams per day
- Pantethine—450 milligrams twice per day
- Plant sterols—2 grams per day
- Red yeast rice—2,400 to 4,800 milligrams per day
- Sesame—40 grams per day
- Soluble fiber—50 grams per day
- Vitamin E—100 milligrams of gamma-/delta-tocotrienols per day

ATTACK PLAN #8: TO LOWER LDL

- EGCG—500 milligrams twice per day
- Krill oil—3 grams per day
- Niacin—500 to 1,000 milligrams per day
- Pantethine—450 milligrams twice per day
- Plant sterols—2 grams per day
- Red yeast rice—2,400 to 4,800 milligrams per day
- Sesame—40 grams per day
- Vitamin E—100 milligrams of gamma-/delta-tocotrienols per day

ATTACK PLAN #9: TO LOWER TRIGLYCERIDES

- Fiber—50 grams of mixed fiber per day
- Krill oil—3 grams per day
- Niacin—500 to 1,000 milligrams per day
- Omega-3 fatty acids—3 to 5 grams per day
- Pantethine—450 milligrams twice per day
- Red yeast rice—2400 to 4800 milligrams per day

ATTACK PLAN #10: TO ALTER SCAVENGER RECEPTOR SIGNALING OF NADPH OXIDASE

This enzyme allows macrophages to ingest modified LDL cholesterol and become foam cells, then induce fatty streaks that increase inflammation. Blocking the enzyme reduces this effect.

- N-acetyl cysteine—500 to 1,000 milligrams twice per day
- Trans-resveratrol—250 to 300 milligrams per day

ATTACK PLAN #11: TO LOWER BLOOD SUGAR

- Biotin—8 milligrams twice per day
- Carnosine—500 milligrams twice per day
- Chromium—800 micrograms per day
- Cinnamon—3 grams twice per day
- EGCG—500 milligrams twice per day
- Magnesium malate chelate—500 milligrams twice per day
- R-lipoic acid—100 milligrams twice per day

ATTACK PLAN # 12: TO LOWER BLOOD PRESSURE (see my book titled *WHAT YOUR DOCTOR MAY NOT TELL YOU ABOUT HYPERTENSION*)

- Cocoa—30 grams dark chocolate per day
- CoQ10—100 milligrams twice per day
- Magnesium—500 to 1,000 milligrams twice per day (Caution: if you have kidney disease, consult with your physician before taking magnesium, for you may not be able to excrete the mineral normally, and it could reach dangerous levels in your blood.)
- Modified DASH II diet
- Omega-3 fatty acids—3 to 5 grams per day
- Potassium—5,000 milligrams per day (Caution: if you have kidney disease, consult with your physician before taking potassium, for you may not be able to excrete the mineral normally, and it could reach dangerous levels in your blood.)
- R-lipoic acid—100 milligrams twice per day
- Sodium—limit to 2,000 milligrams per day
- Taurine—3 grams twice per day

- Trans-resveratrol—250 milligrams once per day
- Vitamin B$_6$—100 milligrams twice per day
- Vitamin C—500 milligrams twice per day
- Vitamin D—increase the blood level to 50–60 ng/mL
- Wakame seaweed—3 to 4 grams per day
- Whey protein—30 grams per day
- Zinc—50 milligrams per day

ATTACK PLAN # 13: TO REDUCE BODY FAT

- Carnitine tartrate powder—2 grams three times per day with meals
- EGCG—500 milligrams twice per day
- Omega-3 fatty acids—5 grams per day or more
- Trans-resveratrol—350 milligrams once per day

Assessing Functional Heart Age

I F YOU ASK a typical patient how old his heart is, he is likely to look a bit baffled as he replies, "As old as I am." He's correct in the sense that his heart and his arteries were born the same moment he was but wrong in the sense that different parts of the body age at different rates. You see this easily with skin: some people in their fifties or sixties have saggy, wrinkled, and blotched skin, while others have firm, plump, and relatively unmarred skin. The differences are due to genetics, sun exposure, diet, weight, exercise, stress, sleep, and more.

The same applies to the heart and the arteries. Chronologically speaking, they are exactly as old as you are, but from a functional point of view, they may be younger or older—and significantly so. As Sir William Osler said, "You are as old as your arteries." Genetics, diet, exercise habits, and numerous other factors speed or slow the aging of the heart and blood vessels, which is why some people enter their senior years in excellent cardiovascular health, while others begin to struggle when they are much younger.

Unfortunately, humans aren't born with a "health dashboard" somewhere on the body that would indicate exactly how the cardiovascular system is doing. The good news is that high-tech tests developed over the past couple of decades can give us a pretty good idea of how the heart and arteries are faring and offer a sense of whether they are functionally younger or older than the number of candles on your birthday cake.

FINDING OUT WHAT'S HAPPENING INSIDE

We don't yet have the testing technology that would allow us to tell exactly how much older or younger than you your heart and arteries are. We can't say, "Mr. Jones, you are fifty-two and your heart is fifty-seven years old," or "Ms. Taylor, your heart is 3.7 years younger than you are." However, we can get a very good idea of whether your heart and arteries are functioning as they should for a person of your age—and knowing that is an important step in protecting and strengthening them and slowing their functional aging if necessary.

We do this by checking for the presence and severity of each of the major risk factors, utilizing new and exciting noninvasive cardiovascular tests that determine the age of your arteries as well as a genetic test called the telomere test that looks at chromosome length to predict biological age. Here is a list of my "top 20" risk factors for coronary heart disease, plus the tests that can be performed for each.

1. Endothelial Dysfunction—Easily measured by several tests performed in the doctor's office. Taking less than fifteen minutes each to complete, they are accurate, noninvasive, and relatively inexpensive. Because they measure endothelial dysfunction and vascular elasticity as well as central blood pressure in the aorta, they have a high predictive value for future cardiovascular diseases such as coronary heart disease, heart attack, stroke, and peripheral artery disease—and also predict arterial age. These tests include the computerized arterial pulse waveform analysis (CAPWA), EndoPAT, digital thermal monitoring (DTM), carotid artery duplex, and ankle-brachial index (ABI).

2. Increased Oxidative Stress and/or Lack of Oxidative Defenses—Measured with blood and urine tests for such markers as 8-hydroxyguanosine (8-OHG), deoxyguanosine (8 OHdG), malondialdehyde (MDA), 8-iso-prostane, catalase, glutathione, SOD (superoxide dismutase), and TBARS, as well as with the oxygen radical antioxidant capacity (ORAC) test and comet assay.

3. Dyslipidemia—Measured with the expanded lipid profiles that go beyond the standard tests for total cholesterol, LDL, HDL, and triglycerides. The expanded lipid profiles include these, plus LDL size and particle number, HDL size and type, VLDL, remnant particles, lipoprotein(a), apolipoprotein B, apolipoprotein C-II, apolipoprotein A-I and A-II, paroxonase, oxLDL, omega-3 index, and serum free fatty acids. It sounds like a lot, but it's all done with a simple blood test, just as if you were having a "regular" cholesterol test. These new expanded lipid profile tests include the LPP (Lipoprotein Particle Profile by SpectraCell Laboratories), NMR (nuclear magnetic resonance by LipoScience), LDL-S_3GGE and HDL-S_{10}GGE (Berkeley Heart Lab), and VAP (Vertical Auto Profile by Atherotec).

4. Increased HS-CRP and Inflammation—Measured by blood tests for HS-CRP, TNF-alpha, interleukin-6, interleukin-1B, and others.

5. Elevated Homocysteine—Measured by blood tests indicating low levels of vitamin B_{12}, vitamin B_6, or folic acid, or a genetic defect in the MTHFR (methylenetetrahydrofolate reductase) gene that contains the code for the MTHFR enzyme.

6. Hypertension—Measured by a number of tests, including twenty-four-hour ambulatory blood pressure monitoring (twenty-four-hour ABM). This is now the "gold standard" test, providing much more information than the standard blood pressure check performed in the doctor's office at a yearly examination. It's also possible to use home blood pressure monitors that have only an upper arm cuff, if patients are instructed on how to use them properly. Wrist and finger blood pressure cuffs are not accurate and should not be used.

Thanks to decades of exciting research, we now know that hypertension is a much more complex disease that we thought it was, caused by a constellation of factors rather than simply consuming too much salt or suffering too much stress. We now understand that hypertension, like coronary heart disease, begins in the arteries and progresses in the following fashion:

1. increased oxidative stress in the blood vessels
2. inflammation of the blood vessels
3. autoimmune dysfunction of the blood vessels
4. abnormal vascular biology with endothelial dysfunction and abnormal vascular smooth muscle

This means hypertension is more than a disease; it's a syndrome that incorporates and interacts with numerous disease states. As Figure 4 shows, hypertension is related to problems in the arteries and kidneys, alterations in the way the body handles blood sugar and fats, changes in the structure and function of the heart, and much more. And once hypertension begins, it contributes to the growth of some of these same harmful states, setting up a bidirectional negative feedback loop that can lead to disaster.

Because hypertension is such as complex disease, a single measurement taken once a year in a doctor's office is not sufficient. Although it will detect obvious cases of high blood pressure, it will fail to identify subtle changes that signal the early stages of hypertension, as well as hypertension that "comes and goes" and may not be present during the minute or two the doctor is taking the yearly reading. Many tests can be used to gauge your cardiovascular health, and they will be discussed in

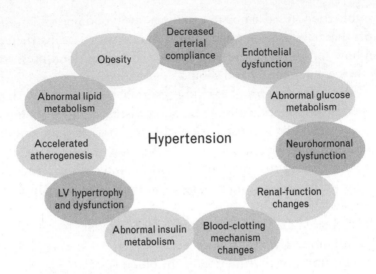

Figure 4: The Hypertension Syndrome Is More Than Just Blood Pressure

the following section. The blood pressure variants that can be evaluated include the following:

- *Dippers and Nondippers*—Blood pressure usually dips (drops) about 10 percent during sleep but should not fall much more. Excessive dipping, reverse dipping, and lack of dipping all indicate problems. These are detected with twenty-four-hour ambulatory blood pressure monitoring.
- *Blood Pressure Variability and Baroreceptor Dysfunction and Sensitivity*—Baroreceptors are small areas of the arteries that monitor blood pressure and signal the brain. Variability in blood pressure is an independent risk factor for heart disease and stroke. Problems with blood variability and baroreceptors can be detected with twenty-four-hour ambulatory blood pressure monitoring.
- *Morning Surges in Blood Pressure*—Blood pressure typically increases early in the morning, even before you get

out of bed, as your body prepares itself for the day. This is part of the circadian rhythm. A safe increase is less than 5 percent. More than a 20-percent increase suggests danger. This is detected with twenty-four-hour ambulatory blood pressure monitoring.

- *Pulse Wave Contour, Augmentation Index, and Pace Wave Velocity (PWV)*—Blood doesn't move through the arteries as a single block; instead, it pulses through, at times rapidly and at times more slowly. When the thrust generated by a single heartbeat nears the end of the vasculature, the energy of the wave is reflected back to the heart. The behavior of the pulse wave changes with age and certain disease states, including endothelial dysfunction. The pulse wave can be monitored via the CAPWA to predict the risk of heart disease and stroke by detecting increased aortic stiffness, augmentation of the systolic pressure, changes in wave reflection, and more.

- *White Coat Hypertension*—This is the tendency of blood pressure to rise when you go to the doctor's office. It is detected with a twenty-four-hour ambulatory blood pressure monitoring or by having the patient measure blood pressure at home, either using a well-standardized automatic cuff or a standard blood pressure cuff and stethoscope.

- *Masked Hypertension*—The opposite of white coat hypertension, this is a drop in usually elevated blood pressure that occurs when a patient goes to the doctor's office for an examination. It is detected with twenty-four-hour ambulatory blood pressure monitoring.

- *Widened Pulse Pressure*—A blood pressure reading is given as two numbers, as in 120/80. The first number, the systolic pressure, is the pressure when the heart is contracting. The second number, the diastolic pressure, is the pressure when the heart is at rest. Subtracting the diastolic (lower number) from the systolic pressure (higher number) produces the pulse pressure, which in this case is 40. A smaller number, showing that the systolic and diastolic readings are narrowly separated, suggests poor heart function, low cardiac output, heart failure, or fluid around the heart (pericardial effusion). A larger number, which occurs when the gap between the systolic and diastolic pressures has widened, indicates the presence of very stiff arteries that have lost their elasticity, which is a sign of atherosclerosis. A widened pulse pressure is detected via a simple calculation after taking the blood pressure. A safe result is usually about 40 to 50.

- *Hypertensive Response to Exercise*—The systolic blood pressure normally increases with exercise, but not much over 180 mm Hg. (The diastolic blood pressure falls or stays the same with exercise.) A systolic pressure that climbs too high or a diastolic pressure that increases at all indicates endothelial dysfunction, loss of arterial elasticity, and a tendency toward future hypertension. It also could indicate extremely poor cardiovascular conditioning. This is detected with a cardiac stress test, as well as with twenty-four-hour ambulatory blood pressure monitoring (if the patient exercises during the twenty-four-hour period). A safe result is a systolic blood pressure less than 180 mm Hg and either no change or about a 10-percent decrease in the diastolic blood pressure.

- *Salt Sensitivity*—Some 10 to 20 percent of Americans are salt sensitive, although among African Americans, the rate can be as much as 75 percent. Salt sensitivity is detected by measuring a blood pressure increase when sodium chloride or table salt is administered or a decrease when salt is restricted. A safe result is usually less than a 10-percent increase in blood pressure with salt administration.

- *Left Ventricular Hypertrophy and Decreased Diastolic Relaxation*—The left ventricle, which is the largest of the four heart chambers, is responsible for propelling freshly oxygenated blood throughout the body. Hypertrophy, or enlargement of the left ventricle, may occur naturally as a result of aerobic training, or it may represent a diseased heart's attempt to compensate for having to pump against increased blood pressure, an abnormal heart value, or intrinsic weakness by growing bigger. Hypertension, for example, can cause the left ventricle to grow larger as it attempts to push the blood through the body against increased resistance. Left ventricular hypertrophy can be measured with echocardiography.

- *Increased Arterial Stiffness*—Arteriosclerosis is the name given to stiffening of the arteries, which may occur for many reasons, including hypertension, dyslipidemia, or diabetes. Stiffened arteries are less able to perform their job, which means blood flow will suffer and produce a variety of symptoms, depending on which parts of the body are affected. If it occurs in the legs, for example, you will have leg cramps on moderate exercise (peripheral artery disease or claudication). Note that arteriosclerosis, or arterial stiffening, is not the same thing as atherosclerosis, which involves the deposition of plaque within the arterial walls. Atherosclerosis is a form of arteriosclerosis. This is detected with the CAPWA.

- *Increased Carotid Intimal-Medial Thickness*—This thickness, which is strongly associated with coronary heart disease and predictive of future cardiovascular disease events, is detected with the carotid intimal-medial thickness (IMT) test.

- *Coronary Calcification*—This is one of the major risk factors that predicts coronary heart disease and future heart attacks—the more calcium present, the greater the risk of suffering a heart attack. Coronary calcification is detected with tests such as electron beam tomography (EBT).

- *Endothelial Dysfunction*—This is detected with the CAPWA, EndoPAT, DTM, and other tests.

- *Microalbuminuria*—This is detected with the spot urine test.

- *Elevated Creatinine and Reduced GFR*—Creatinine is a breakdown product of muscle that is normally removed from the blood by the kidneys. When the kidneys are performing poorly, the creatinine level rises. The glomerular filtration rate (GFR) measures kidney function and helps assess the extent of kidney disease. The creatinine level is measured with a blood test, and the result is used to calculate the GFR. A normal creatinine level is below 1.0 mg, and a normal GFR is over 100 cc per minute.

- *Hypertensive Retinopathy*—Briefly put, this is damage to the retina, the back part of the eye, caused by elevated blood pressure. Using an ophthalmoscope or other special retinal imaging device, a doctor can see narrowing of the blood vessels in the retina, indentations, atherosclerosis, and other problems. The retinal arteries are considered to be a "window" to the arteries in the brain, and thus to the arteries in the body, allowing us to assess their condition by simply looking in the eye. The retinal arteries should not be small, thickened, or indented.

- *Elevated HS-CRP*—This is detected with blood tests for HS-CRP. A normal value is less than 2.0 mg/dL.

- *Elevated Central Blood Pressure (CBP)*—Most people think that a blood pressure reading can measure only the peripheral pressure, or pressure in the upper arm, but it's possible to detect the pressure in the ascending aorta, the large artery rising up out of the heart. This is the central blood pressure—the pressure of the blood as it leaves the heart—which is a better predictor of cardiovascular disease and left ventricular hypertrophy than the standard blood pressure reading. Directly measuring central blood pressure is an invasive procedure that requires threading a pressure sensor from an artery in the groin into the aorta. However, central pressure can also be indirectly determined using noninvasive blood pressure/cardiovascular machines to detect the blood pressure at different points on the body and the differences between them. This information is plugged into a mathematical formula that produces central blood pressure readings. The central pressure should be about 120/80 mm Hg or less.

- *Peripheral Artery Disease*—Problems caused by poor blood flow in the legs may be detected with the ABI.

It's not necessary to perform all of these tests to determine your cardiovascular risk. However, it is important to measure your blood pressure more than once per year and to have a twenty-four-hour ambulatory blood pressure monitor to avoid improper diagnosis, overtreatment, or undertreatment. It's best to invest the additional time and money to either be assured that your pressure is within the safe range or to detect and begin treating problems early.

7. Biological Age—This is determined within five years or less using a telomere test to determine telomere length. Longer telomeres indicate a reduced risk of heart disease and predict slower vascular aging and slower aging in general. The telomere test is available from SpectraCell Laboratories in Houston, Texas.

8. "Dangerous" Genetics—Can be detected with SNP testing. Genetic alterations that can cause obvious and serious blood pressure and cardiac problems include the ACE D/D and I/D genes, the adducin gene, and the angiotensinogen gene. However, many of us have other changes in our genes called SNPs that act very subtly, predisposing us to diseases that strike only when other factors come into play.

SNP stands for single nucleotide polymorphism, which is a small genetic alteration in the DNA that occurs when one of the four "letters" that make up the genetic alphabet—the nucleotides known as adenine (A), cytosine (C), thymine (T), and guanine (G)—is replaced by one of the other letters. For example, perhaps the sequence of "letters" in a segment of DNA should be ACTTCAG—but instead, the last "letter" is changed, and it becomes ACTTCAT. That's a single nucleotide polymorphism, or SNP.

SNPs are common, and many are inconsequential. However, if they occur within a portion of the DNA that codes for a protein, they can change the way that protein behaves. This altered protein may not be deformed enough to trigger disease on its own, but if it changes the way the body converts nutrients from one form to another, the way it processes blood sugar, or the way it performs thousands of other actions, it may tip the balance in favor of disease. Suppose, for example, a certain SNP makes it a little bit harder for the body to metabolize vitamin D. It won't matter to people who consume plenty of the vitamin or make their own when their skin is exposed to sunlight. But if this SNP occurs in a person whose diet is low in vitamin D, who lives in a cloudy climate and is not exposed to much sunlight, and takes antacids and other medicines that interfere with vitamin D, the risk of a vitamin D deficiency disease increases dramatically. In other words, the SNP creates a small weakness that may be converted into a major problem by diet, lack of physical activity, and other lifestyle factors.

Some SNPs have broad effects on the body, while others can produce specific problems (if lifestyle factors fall into place). For example, a certain SNP on chromosome 1p13 affects the secretion of LDL and increases the risk of suffering a heart attack. Another SNP increases the risk of coronary heart disease by interfering with SOD, a major scavenger of oxygen in the form of O_2, which causes oxidative damage. A "missense" mutation of EC-SOD (R213G) reduces arterial wall SOD and increases plasma SOD. This reduces oxidative defenses in the arterial walls and increases oxidative stress, increasing the risk of coronary heart disease.

More than seven hundred SNPs have been associated with heart disease, hypertension, and cardiovascular health. Here are a few examples of them:

- *Hypertension*—more than five hundred SNPs, including ACE DD, adducin, angiotensinogen, NOS3 ADM, ADRB2, and AGT/M235T
- *HDL and LDL*—PPARc/Pro12A1a, CETP/Tagl, LPL/1595C>G, APOC3/2854T>G, and APO AI/75G>A
- *Oxidative stress and defenses*—SOD2, SOD 3, NOS3, catalase, GPx, and glutathione
- *Inflammation markers*—TNF-alpha, IL-6, IL-1-B
- *Folic acid*—MTHFR
- *Coronary heart disease and heart attack*—EC-SOD, metallothioneins MT1A, CDT, GPx, APO E 4, TSP 1 and 4, YKL-40, KIF 6, CETP TAQ 1B

Don't worry about "translating" the abbreviations above into regular English. The point is that hundreds of SNPs interfere with the healthy functioning of the body and set the stage for coronary heart disease and related ailments. More SNPs remain to be identified and the risks they pose outlined. In the meantime, you can be tested for SNPs that may set you on the path toward coronary heart disease at laboratories such as Doctor's Data, Genova Diagnostics, and Quest Labs.

Remember, however, that a SNP is a predisposition, not a disaster written in stone. Knowing where you have weaknesses can be a blessing, for it allows you to take corrective action.

9. *Calcification Seen on Heart Scans*—Measured by electron beam tomography, a cardiac CT scan, and/or an MRI of the heart.

10. *Hormonal Deficiencies*—Measured by blood, urine, and saliva tests for DHEA, free testosterone, sex hormone binding globulin, estradiol, estriol, estrone, progesterone hormone metabolites, growth hormone, IGF1, and IGF3.

11. *Diabetes Mellitus*—Measured by elevated blood sugar (fasting and after meals), increased insulin and proinsulin levels, C-peptide, hemoglobin A1c, and metabolic syndrome glucose parameters of glucose intolerance.

12. *Hypothyroidism, or Subclinical Disease with Increased Thyroid-Stimulating Hormone (TSH)*—Measured by blood tests for TSH, free T4, free T3, reverse T3, and thyroid antibodies.

13. *Increased Levels of Heavy Metals*—Levels of mercury, lead, cadmium, arsenic, iron, and other metals can be measured via blood and urine tests.

14. *Lack of Exercise*—No test necessary.

15. *Lack of Sleep*—Monitored with sleep studies conducted in special facilities. The patient is hooked up to various monitors and spends the night in the facility as brain waves and other functions are monitored. These are analyzed to determine whether the sleeping problem is organic or has to do with poor sleep hygiene, such as drinking caffeine too soon before bedtime or not darkening the bedroom enough.

16. *Low Vitamin K and Vitamin D Levels*—Measured with standard blood tests.

17. *Left Ventricular Hypertrophy (LVH) and Diastolic Dysfunction (DD)*—Can be seen using an echocardiogram of the heart, as well as other cardiac tests.

18. *Microalbuminuria and/or Kidney Disease*—Identified with blood tests. Microalbuminuria is found with the spot urine test. Kidney disease is detected with a blood test measuring

serum creatinine or calculating the GFR, which determines the stage of kidney disease.

19. Obesity—Measured by calculating and comparing weight, BMI, waist circumference, and a body composition test, which measures both visceral (belly) fat and total body fat.

20. Smoking—No test necessary, for the patient knows if he or she smokes. Direct use of any tobacco product counts, as does indirect, passive smoke inhalation caused by being around smokers in a smoky environment.

Resources

Recommended Companies and Labs

Educational Organizations

The Institute for Functional Medicine (IFM)
4411 Pt. Fosdick Drive NW, Suite 305
PO Box 1697
Gig Harbor, WA 98335
Web: www.functionalmedicine.org
Phone: 800-228-0622, 253-858-4724
Fax: 253-853-6766

The American Academy of Anti-Aging on Regenerative
Medicine (A4M)
1801 North Military Trail, Suite 200
Boca Raton, FL 33431
Web: www.a4m.com
Email: info@a4m.com
Phone: 888-997-0112
Fax: 561-997-0287

Nutrition Companies

Biotics Research Corporation
6801 Biotics Research Drive
Rosenberg, TX 77471

Web: www.bioticsresearch.com
Email: biotics@bioticsresearch.com
Phone: 800-231-5777
Fax: 281-344-0725

Designs for Health
980 South Street
Suffield, CT 06078
Web: www.designsforhealth.com
Email: orders@designsforhealth.com
Phone: 800-367-4325
Fax: 206-333-0408

AC Grace
111 East Gilmer Street
PO Box 570
Big Sandy, TX 75755
Web: www.acgrace.com
Phone: 800-833-4368
Fax: 903-636-4051

Testing Companies

SpectraCell Laboratories (Micronutrient Test,
    LPP expanded lipid profile, and Telomere Test)
10401 Town Park Drive
Houston, TX 77072
Web: www.spectracell.com
Email: spec1@spectracell.com
Phone: 800-227-5227 or 713-621-3101
Fax: 713-621-3234

Hypertension Diagnostics: HDI Profiler (CAPWA)
2915 Waters Road, Suite 108
Eagan, MN 55121
Web: www.hdii.com

Email: infoteam@hdii.com
Phone: 888-PulseWave (785-7392)
Fax: 651-687-0485

Itamar Medical: EndoPAT
842 Upper Union Street, Suite 2
Franklin, MA 02038
Web: www.intamar-medical.com
Email: infousa@itamar-medical.com
Phone: 888-748-2627
Fax: 888-748-2628

HeartSmart Carotic IMT
19700 Fairchild
Irvine, CA 92612
Email: info@heartsmart.com
Phone: 949-724-1700

EXERCISE AND PERFORMANCE CENTERS

Poliquin Performance Centers and Headquarters
42 Ladd Street #109
East Greenwich, RI 02818
Email: info@charlespoliquin.com
Phone: 401-398-7845, 855-398-7845 (toll-free)
Fax: 401-398-7160

Notes

Chapter Three: A Fast Track to Heart Disease

1. El Fadi, K.A., N. Ragy, M. El Batran, et al. "Periodontitis and Cardiovascular Disease: Floss and Reduce a Potential Risk Factor for CVD." *Angiology* 2010 Aug 3. [Epub ahead of print].

2. Schmelzer, C., I. Lindner, G. Rimbach, et al. "Functions of Coenzyme Q10 in Inflammation and Gene Expression." *Biofactors* 2008; 32(1–4):179–183.

3. Wang X.L., D.L. Rainwater, C. Mahaney, R. Stocker. "Cosupplementation with Vitamin E and Coenzyme Q10 Reduces Circulating Markers of Inflammation in Baboons." *American Journal of Clinical Nutrition* 2004; 80(3):649–655.

4. Kadoglou, N.P., F. Iliadis, N. Angelopoulou, et al. "The Antiinflammatory Effects of Exercise Training in Patients with Type 2 Diabetes." *European Journal of Cardiovascular Prevention and Rehabilitation* 2007; 14(6):837–843.

5. See, for example, Donges, C.E., R. Duffield, and E.J. Drinkwater. "Effects of Resistance or Aerobic Exercise Training on Interleukin-6, C-Reactive Protein, and Body Composition." *Medicine and Science in Sports and Exercise* 2010; 42(2):304–313.

6. Murakami, K., S. Sasaki, Y. Takahashi, et al. "Total n-3 Polyunsaturated Fatty Acid Intake Is Inversely Associated with Serum C-Reactive Protein in Young Japanese Women." *Nutrition Research* 2008; 28(5):309–314.

7. Block G., C.D. Jensen, T.B. Dalvi, et al. "Vitamin C Treatment Reduces Elevated C-Reactive Protein." *Free Radical Biology and Medicine* 2009; 46(1):70–77.

Chapter Four: Quenching Oxidation, a Disaster in the Making

1. Blankenberg, S., H.J. Rupprecht, C. Bickel, et al. "Glutathione Peroxidase 1 Activity and Cardiovascular Events in Patients with Coronary Artery Disease." *New England Journal of Medicine* 2003; 349(17):1605–1613.

2. Hninger, I., M. Chopra, D.I. Thurnham, et al. "Effect of Increased Fruit and Vegetable Intake on the Susceptibility of Lipoprotein to Oxidation in Smokers." *European Journal of Clinical Nutrition* 1997; 51(9):601–606.

3. Southon, S. "Increased Fruit and Vegetable Consumption: Potential Health Benefits." *Nutrition, Metabolism, and Cardiovascular Diseases* 2001; 11(4 Suppl):78–81.

4. Roberts, W.G., M.H. Gordon, A.F. Walker. "Effects of Enhanced Consumption of Fruit and Vegetables on Plasma Antioxidant Status and Oxidative Resistance of LDL in Smokers Supplemented with Fish Oil." *European Journal of Clinical Nutrition* 2003; 57(10):1303–1310.

5. M.C. Houston et al. "Juice Powder Concentrate and Systemic Blood Pressure, Progression of Coronary Artery Calcium and Antioxidant Status in Hypertensive Subjects: A Pilot Study." *Evidenced-Based Complementary and Alternative Medicine* 2007; 4:455–462.

6. Coimbra, S., E. Castro, P. Rocha-Pereira, et al. "The Effect of Green Tea in Oxidative Stress." *Clinical Nutrition* 2006; 25(5): 790–796.

7. Young, J.F., L.O. Dragstedt, J. Haraldsdottir, et al. "Green Tea Extract Only Affects Markers of Oxidative Status Postprandially: Lasting Antioxidant Effect of Flavonoid-Free Diet." *British Journal of Nutrition* 2002; 87(4):343–355.

Chapter Five: Fixing Cholesterol: Beyond the Numbers

1. The levels of the items in this and the next two bulleted items can be measured by one of the new expanded lipid profile tests, such as Lipoprotein Particle Profile (LPP) by SpectraCell Laboratories, nuclear magnetic resonance (NMR) by LipoScience, LDL-S_3GGE and HDL-S_{10}GGE by Berkeley Heart Lab, or Vertical Auto Profile (VAP) by Atherotec.

2. Salmeron, J., F.B. Hu, J.E. Manson, et al. "Dietary Fat Intake and Risk of Type 2 Diabetes in Women." *American Journal of Clinical Nutrition* 2001; 73(6):1019–1026. Lichtenstein, A.H., L.M. Ausman, S.M. Jalbert, et al. "Effects of Different Forms of Dietary Hydrogenated Fats on Serum Lipoprotein Cholesterol Levels." *New England Journal of Medicine* 1999; 340(25):1933–1940. Lemaitre, R.N., I.B. King, T.E. Raghunathan, et al. "Cell Membrane Trans Fatty Acids and the Risk of Primary Cardiac Arrest." *Circulation* 2002; 105(6):697–701. Oomen, C.M., M.C. Ocke, E.J. Feskens, et al. "Association Between Trans Fatty Acid Intake and 10-Year Risk of Coronary Heart Disease in the Zutphen Elderly Study: A Prospective Population-Based Study." *Lancet* 2001; 357(9258):746–751. Schaefer, E.J. "Lipoprotein, Nutrition, and Heart Disease." *American Journal of Clinical Nutrition* 2002; 75(2):191–212.

3. Raederstorff, D.G., M.F. Schlacter, V. Elste, et al. "Effect of EGCG on Lipid Absorption and Plasma Lipid Levels in Rats." *Journal of Nutritional Biochemistry* 2003; 14(6):326–332. Lin, J.K., and S.Y. Lin-Shiau. "Mechanisms of Hypolipidemic and Anti-Obesity Effects of Tea and Tea Polyphenols." *Molecular Nutrition and Food Research* 2006; 50(2):211–217. Hirano-Ohmori, R., R. Takahashi, Y. Momiyama, et al. "Green Tea Consumption and Serum Malondialdehyde-Modified LDL Concentrations in Healthy Subjects." *Journal of the American College of Nutrition* 2005; 24(5): 342–346. Erba, D., P. Riso, A. Bordoni, et al. "Effectiveness of Moderate Green Tea Consumption on Antiioxidative Status and Plasma Lipid Profile in Humans." *Journal of Nutritional Biochemistry* 2005; 16(3):144–149. Tokunaga S, I.R. White, C. Frost, et al. "Green Tea Consumption and Serum Lipids and Lipoproteins in a Population

of Healthy Workers in Japan." *Annals of Epidemiology* 2002; 12(3): 157–165. Singha, D.K., S. Banerjeeb, T.D. Portera, et al. "Green and Black Tea Extracts Inhibit HMG-CoA Reductase and Activate AMP Kinase to Decrease Cholesterol Synthesis in Hepatoma Cells." *Journal of Nutritional Biochemistry* 2009; 20(10):816–822.

4. Wu, S.J., P.L. Liu, L.T. Ng. "Tocotrienol-Rich Fraction of Palm Oil Exhibits Anti-inflammatory Property by Suppressing the Expression of Inflammatory Mediators in Human Monocytic Cells." *Molecular Nutrition and Food Research* 2008; 52(8):921–929. Das, S., K. Nesaretnam, D.K. Das. "Tocotrienols in Cardioprotection." *Vitamins and Hormones* 2007; 76:419–433.

5. Wittwer, C.T., C.P. Graves, M.A. Peterson, et al. "Pantethine Lipomodulation: Evidence for Cysteamine Mediation in Vitro and in Vivo." *Atherosclerosis* 1987; 68(1–2):41–49. Cighetti, G., M. Del Puppo, R. Paroni, et al. "Modulation of HMG-CoA Reductase Activity by Pantetheine/Pantethine." *Biochimica et Biophysica Acta* 1988; 963(2):389–393.

Chapter Six: Maintaining Proper Blood Flow Through the Arteries

1. Sankar, D., M.R. Rao, G. Sambandam, K.V. Pugalendi. "A Pilot Study of Open Label Sesamin Oil in Hypertensive Diabetics." *Journal of Medicinal Food* 2006; 9(3):408–412.

2. "McDonald's USA Nutrition Facts for Popular Menu Items," effective date April 6, 2011. Accessible at http://nutrition.mcdonalds .com/nutritionexchange/nutritionfacts.pdf. Viewed May 14, 2011.

Chapter Seven: Preventing Blood Sugar and Insulin from Harming the Heart

1. Sankar, D., M.R. Rao, G. Sambandam, K.V. Pugalendi. "A Pilot Study of Open Label Sesamin Oil in Hypertensive Diabetics." *Journal of Medicinal Food* 2006; 9(3):408–412.

2. Cefalu, W.T., and F.B. Hu. "Role of Chromium in Human Health and in Diabetes." *Diabetes Care* 2004; 27(11):2741–2751.

3. Iso, H., C. Date, K. Wakai, et al. "The Relationship Between Green Tea and Total Caffeine Intake and Risk for Self-Reported Type 2 Diabetes Among Japanese Adults." *Annals of Internal Medicine* 2006; 144(8):554–562.

4. Oh, C.J., E.S. Yang, S.W. Shin, et al. "Epigallocatechin Gallate, a Constituent of Green Tea, Regulates High Glucose-Induced Apoptosis." *Archives of Pharmaceutical Research* 2008; 31(1):34–40.

Chapter Eight: A Potpourri of Other Risk Factors

1. Offered by SpectraCell Laboratories of Houston, Texas.

2. Ruiz, J.R., X. Sui, F. Lobelo, et al. "Association Between Muscular Strength and Mortality in Men: Prospective Cohort Study." *British Medical Journal* 2008; 337(7661):92–95.

3. Eguchi, K., S. Hoshide, S. Ishikawa, et al. "Short Sleep Duration Is an Independent Predictor of Stroke Events in Elderly Hypertensive Patients." *Journal of the American Society of Hypertension* 2010; 4(5):255–262.

Appendix III: Quenching Inflammation and Controlling High-Sensitivity C-Reactive Protein

1. Ahluwalia, N., A. Genoux, J. Ferrieres, et al. "Iron Status Is Associated with Carotid Atherosclerotic Plaques in Middle-Aged Adults." *Journal of Nutrition* 2010; 149(4):812–816.

2. Depalma, R.G., V.W. Hayes, B.K. Chow, et al. "Ferritin Levels, Inflammatory Biomarkers, and Mortality in Peripheral Arterial Disease: A Substudy of the Iron (Fe) and Atherosclerosis Study (FeAST) Trial." *Journal of Vascular Surgery* 2010; 51(6): 1498–1503.

3. El Fadi, K.A., N. Ragy, M. El Batran, et al. "Periodontitis and Cardiovascular Disease: Floss and Reduce a Potential Risk Factor for CVD." *Angiology* 2010; 62(1):62–67.

4. Esposito, K., R. Marfella, M. Ciotola, et al. "Effect of a Mediterranean-Style Diet on Endothelial Dysfunction and Markers of Vascular Inflammation in the Metabolic Syndrome: A

Randomized Trial." *Journal of the American Medical Association* 2004; 292(12):1440–1446.

5. Blum, S., M. Aviram, A. Ben-Amotz, Y. Levy. "Effect of a Mediterranean Meal on Postprandial Carotenoids, Paraoxonase Activity and C-Reactive Protein." *Annals of Nutrition and Metabolism* 2006; 50(1):20–24.

6. Adamsson, V., A. Reumark, I.B. Fredriksson, E. Hammarstrom, et al. "Effects of a Healthy Nordic Diet on Cardiovascular Risk Factors in Hypercholesterolaemic Subjects: A Randomized Controlled Trial (NORDIET)." *Journal of Internal Medicine* 2010; Sep 28. doi:10.111/j. [Epub ahead of print].

7. Oliveira, A., F. Rodriguez-Artalego, C. Lopes. "The Association of Fruits, Vegetables, Antioxidant Vitamins and Fibre Intake with High-Sensitivity C-Reactive Protein: Sex and Body Mass Index Interactions." *European Journal of Clinical Nutrition.* 2009; 63(11):1345–1352.

8. Micallef, M.A., I.A. Munro, M.L. Garg. "An Inverse Relationship Between Plasma n-3 Fatty Acids and C-Reactive Protein in Healthy Individuals." *European Journal of Clinical Nutrition* 2009; 63(9):1154–1156.

9. Murakami, K., S. Sasaki, Y. Takahashi, et al. "Total n-3 Polyunsaturated Fatty Acid Intake Is Inversely Associated with Serum C-Reactive Protein in Young Japanese Women." *Nutrition Research* 2008; 28(5):309–314.

10. Burr, M.L., A.M. Fehily, J.F. Gilbert, et al. "Effects of Changes in Fat, Fish, and Fibre Intakes on Death and Myocardial Reinfarction: Diet and Reinfarction Trial (DART)." *Lancet* 1989; 2(8666):757–761.

11. Micallef, M.A. and M.L. Garg. "Anti-Inflammatory and Cardioprotective Effects of n-3 Polyunsaturated Fatty Acids and Plant Sterols in Hyperlipidemic Individuals." *Atherosclerosis* 2009; 204(2):476–482.

12. Brighenti, F., S. Valtuene, N. Pellegrini, et al. "Total Antioxidant Capacity of the Diet Is Inversely and Independently Related to Plasma Concentration of High-Sensitivity C-Reactive Protein in Adult Italian Subjects." *British Journal of Nutrition* 2005; 93(5):619–625.

13. Sato, K., Y. Dohi, M. Kojima, et al. "Effects of Ascorbic Acid on Ambulatory Blood Pressure in Elderly Patients with Refractory Hypertension." *Arzneimittelforschung* 2006; 56(7):535–540.

14. Block, G., C.D. Jensen, T.B. Dalvi, et al. "Vitamin C Treatment Reduces Elevated C-Reactive Protein." *Free Radical Biology and Medicine* 2009; 46(1):70–77.

15. Chacko, S.A., Y. Song, L. Nathan, et al. "Relations of Dietary Magnesium Intake to Biomarkers of Inflammation and Endothelial Dysfunction in an Ethnically Diverse Cohort of Postmenopausal Women." *Diabetes Care* 2010; 33(2):304–310.

16. Ridker, P.M., M. Cushman, M.J. Stampfer, et al. "Inflammation, Aspirin, and the Risk of Cardiovascular Disease in Apparently Healthy Men." *New England Journal of Medicine,* 1997; 336(14):973–979.

17. Kronish, I.M., N. Rieckmann, D. Shimbo, et al. "Aspirin Adherence, Aspirin Dosage, and C-Reactive Protein in the First Three Months After Acute Coronary Syndrome." *American Journal of Cardiology* 2010; 106(8):1090–1094.

18. Qi, L., R.M. van Dam, S. Kiu, et al. "Whole-Grain, Bran, and Cereal Fiber Intakes and Markers of Systemic Inflammation in Diabetic Women." *Diabetes Care* 2006, 29(2):207–211.

19. Gentile, M., S. Panico, F. Rubba, et al. "Obesity, Overweight, and Weight Gain Over Adult Life Are Main Determinants of Elevated HS-CRP in a Cohort of Mediterranean Women." *European Journal of Clinical Nutrition* 2010; 64(8):873–878.

20. Aeberli, I., L. Molinari, G. Spinas, et al. "Dietary Intakes of Fat and Antioxidant Vitamins Are Predictors of Subclinical Inflammation in Overweight Swiss Children." *American Journal of Clinical Nutrition* 2006; 84(4):748–755.

21. Kadoglou, N.P., F. Iliadis, N. Angelopoulou, et al. "The Anti-Inflammatory Effects of Exercise Training in Patients with Type 2 Diabetes." *European Journal of Cardiovascular Prevention and Rehabilitation* 2007; 14(6):837–843.

22. See, for example, Donges, C.E., R. Duffield, E.J. Drinkwater. "Effects of Resistance or Aerobic Exercise Training on Interleukin-6, C-Reactive Protein, and Body Composition." *Medicine and Science in Sports and Exercise* 2010; 42(2):304–313.

23. Hale, L.P., P.K. Greer, G.D. Sempowski. "Bromelain Treatment Alters Leukocyte Expression of Cell Surface Molecules Involved in Cellular Adhesion and Activation." *Clinical Immunology* 2002; 104(2):183–190.

24. Monagas, M., N. Khan, C. Andres-Lacueva, et al. "Effect of Cocoa Powder on the Modulation of Inflammatory Biomarkers in Patients at High Risk of Cardiovascular Disease." *American Journal of Clinical Nutrition* 2009; 90(5):1144–1150.

25. Wang, X.L., D.L. Rainwater, C. Mahaney, R. Stocker. "Cosupplementation with Vitamin E and Coenzyme Q10 Reduces Circulating Markers of Inflammation in Baboons." *American Journal of Clinical Nutrition* 2004; 80(3):649–655.

26. Schmelzer, C., I. Lindner, G. Rimbach, et al. "Functions of Coenzyme Q10 in Inflammation and Gene Expression." *Biofactors* 2008; 32(1–4):179–183.

27. Melgarejo, E., M.A. Medina, F. Sanchez-Jimenez, J.L. Urdiales. "Epigallocatechin Gallate Reduces Human Monocyte Mobility and Adhesion in Vitro." *British Journal of Pharmacology* 2009; 158(7):1705–1712.

28. Yamakuchi, M., C. Bao, M. Ferlito, C.J. Lowenstein. "Epigallocatechin Gallate Inhibits Endothelial Exocytosis." *Journal of Biological Chemistry* 2008; 389(7):935–941.

29. Mink, P.J., C.G. Scafford, L.M. Barraj, et al. "Flavonoid Intake and Cardiovascular Disease Mortality: A Prospective Study in Postmenopausal Women." *American Journal of Clinical Nutrition* 2007; 85(3):895–909.

30. Belcaro, G., M.R. Cesarone, S. Errichi, et al. "Variations in C-Reactive Protein, Plasma Free Radicals and Fibrinogen Values in Patients with Osteoarthritis Treated with Pycnogenol." *Redox Report* 2008; 13(6):271–276.

31. Walker, A.F., G. Marakis, E. Simpson, et al. "Hypotensive Effects of Hawthorn for Patients with Diabetes Taking Prescription Drugs: A Randomised Controlled Trial." *British Journal of General Practice* 2006; 56(527):437–443.

32. Sola, S., M.Q. Mir, F.A. Cheerna, et al. "Irbesartan and Lipoic Acid Improve Endothelial Function and Reduce Markers of

Inflammation in the Metabolic Syndrome: Results of the Irbesartan and Lipoic Acid in Endothelial Dysfunction (ISLAND) Study." *Circulation* 2005; 111(3):343-348.

Appendix IV: Reducing Oxidative Stress

1. Roberts, W.G., M.H. Gordon, A.F. Walker. "Effects of Enhanced Consumption of Fruit and Vegetables on Plasma Antioxidant Status and Oxidative Resistance of LDL in Smokers Supplemented with Fish Oil." *European Journal of Clinical Nutrition* 2003; 57(10):1303-1310.

2. Houston, M., et al. "Juice Powder Concentrate and Systemic Blood Pressure, Progression of Coronary Artery Calcium and Antioxidant Status in Hypertensive Subjects: A Pilot Study." *Evidenced-Based Complementary and Alternative Medicine* 2007; 4:455-462.

3. Coimbra, S., E. Castro, P. Rocha-Pereira, et al. "The Effect of Green Tea in Oxidative Stress. *Clinical Nutrition* 2006; 25(5): 790-796.

4. Young, J.F., L.O. Dragstedt, J. Haraldsdottir, et al. "Green Tea Extract Only Affects Markers of Oxidative Status Postprandially: Lasting Antioxidant Effect of Flavonoid-Free Diet." *British Journal of Nutrition* 2002; 87(4):343-355.

5. Kedziora-Kornatowska, K., K. Szewczyk-Golec, M. Kozakiewicz, et al. "Melatonin Improves Oxidative Stress Parameters Measured in the Blood of Elderly Type 2 Diabetic Patients." *Journal of Pineal Research* 2009; 46(3):333-337.

6. Blankenberg, S., H.J. Rupprecht, C. Bickel, et al. "Glutathione Peroxidase 1 Activity and Cardiovascular Events in Patients with Coronary Artery Disease." *New England Journal of Medicine* 2003; 349(17):1605-1613.

7. Southon, S. "Increased Fruit and Vegetable Consumption: Potential Health Benefits." *Nutrition, Metabolism, and Cardiovascular Disease* 2001; 11(4 Suppl):78-81.

8. Hninger, I., M. Chopra, D.I. Thurnham, et al. "Effect of Increased Fruit and Vegetable Intake on the Susceptibility of

Lipoprotein to Oxidation in Smokers." *European Journal of Clinical Nutrition* 1997; 51(9):601–606.

Appendix V: Antioxidant and Anti-inflammatory Supplements and Other Approaches

1. Salmeron, J., F.B. Hu, J.E. Manson, et al. "Dietary Fat Intake and Risk of Type 2 Diabetes in Women." *American Journal of Clinical Nutrition* 2001; 73(6):1019–1026. Lichtenstein, A.H., L.M. Ausman, S.M. Jalbert, et al. "Effects of Different Forms of Dietary Hydrogenated Fats on Serum Lipoprotein Cholesterol Levels." *New England Journal of Medicine* 1999; 340(25):1933–1940. Lemaitre, R.N., I.B. King, T.E. Raghunathan, et al. "Cell Membrane Trans-Fatty Acids and the Risk of Primary Cardiac Arrest." *Circulation* 2002; 105(6):697–701. Oomen, C.M., M.C. Ocke, E.J. Feskens, et al. "Association Between Trans Fatty Acid Intake and 10-year Risk of Coronary Heart Disease in the Zutphen Elderly Study: A Prospective Population-Based Study." *Lancet* 2001; 357(9258):746–751. Schaefer, E.J. "Lipoprotein, Nutrition, and Heart Disease." *American Journal of Clinical Nutrition* 2002; 75(2):191–212.

2. Wu, W.H., Y.P. Kang, N.H. Wang, et al. "Sesame Ingestion Affects Sex Hormones, Antioxidant Status, and Blood Lipids in Postmenopausal Women." *Journal of Nutritional Science and Vitaminology (Tokyo)* 2006; 136(5):1270–1275.

3. Sankar, D., M.R. Rao, G. Sambandam, K.V. Pugalendi. "A Pilot Study of Open Label Sesamin Oil in Hypertensive Diabetics." *Journal of Medicinal Food* 2006; 9(3):408–412.

4. Miyawaki, T., H. Aono, Y. Toyoda-Ona, et al. "Antihypertensive Effects of Sesamin in Humans." *Journal of Nutritional Science and Vitaminology (Tokyo)* 2009; 55(1):87–91.

5. Harikumar, K.B., B. Sung, S.T. Tharakan, et al. "Sesamin Manifests Chemopreventive Effects Through the Suppression of NF-Kappa B-Regulated Cell Survival, Proliferation, Invasion, and Angiogenic Gene Products." *Molecular Cancer Research* 2010; 8(5):751–761.

6. Raederstorff, D.G., M.F. Schlacter, V. Elste, et al. "Effect of EGCG on Lipid Absorption and Plasma Lipid Levels in Rats." *Journal*

of Nutritional Biochemistry 2003; 14(6):326–332. Lin, J.K. and S.Y. Lin-Shiau. "Mechanisms of Hypolipidemic and Anti-Obesity Effects of Tea and Tea Polyphenols." *Molecular Nutrition and Food Research* 2006; 50(2): 211–217. Hirano-Ohmori, R., R. Takahashi, Y. Momiyama, et al. "Green Tea Consumption and Serum Malondialdehyde-Modified LDL Concentrations in Healthy Subjects." *Journal of the American College of Nutrition* 2005; 24(5): 342–346. Erba, D., P. Riso, A. Bordoni, et al. "Effectiveness of Moderate Green Tea Consumption on Antioxidative Status and Plasma Lipid Profile in Humans." *Journal of Nutritional Biochemistry* 2005; 16(3): 144–149. Tokunaga, S., I.R. White, C. Frost, et al. "Green Tea Consumption and Serum Lipids and Lipoproteins in a Population of Healthy Workers in Japan." *Annals of Epidemiology* 2002; 12(3):157–165. Singha, D.K., S. Banerjeeb, T.D. Portera, et al. "Green and Black Tea Extracts Inhibit HMG-Coa Reductase and Activate AMP Kinase to Decrease Cholesterol Synthesis in Hepatoma Cells." *Journal of Nutritional Biochemistry* 2009; 20(10): 816–822.

7. Mozaffarian, D., and E.B. Rimm. "Fish Intake, Contaminants, and Human Health: Evaluating the Risk and the Benefits." *Journal of the American Medical Association* 2006; 296(15):1885–1899.

8. Farzaneh-Far, R., J. Lin, E.S. Epel, et al. "Association of Marine Omega-3 Fatty Acid Levels with Telomeric Aging in Patients with Coronary Heart Disease." *Journal of the American Medical Association* 2010; 303(3):250–257.

9. Grouilette, S.W., J.S. Moore, A.D. McMahon, et al. "Telomere Length, Risk of Coronary Heart Disease, and Statin Treatment in the West of Scotland Primary Prevention Study: A Nested Case-Control Study." *Lancet* 2007; 369(9556):107–114.

10. The Coronary Drug Project Research Group. "Clofibrate and Niacin in Coronary Heart Disease." *Journal of the American Medical Association* 1975; 231:360–381.

11. Qureshi, A.A., S.S. Sami, W.A. Salser, F.A. Khan. "Dose-Dependent Suppression of Serum Cholesterol by Tocotrienol-Rich Fraction (TRF25) of Rice Bran in Hypercholesterolemic Humans." *Atherosclerosis* 2002; 161(1):199–207.

12. Wu, S.J., P.L. Liu, L.T. Ng. "Tocotrienol-Rich Fraction of Palm Oil Exhibits Anti-Inflammatory Property by Suppressing the Expression of Inflammatory Mediators in Human Monocytic Cells." *Molecular Nutrition and Food Research.* 2008; 52(8):921–929. Das, S., K. Nesaretnam, D.K. Das. "Tocotrienols in Cardioprotection." *Vitamins and Hormones* 2007; 76:419–433.

13. Wittwer, C.T., C.P. Graves, M.A. Peterson, et al. "Pantethine Lipomodulation: Evidence for Cysteamine Mediation in Vitro and in Vivo." *Atherosclerosis* 1987; 68(1–2):41–49. Cighetti, G., M. Del Puppo, R. Paroni, et al. "Modulation of HMG-CoA Reductase Activity by Pantetheine/Pantethine." *Biochimica et Biophysica Acta* 1988; 963(2):389–393.

14. Blair, S.N., D.M. Capuzzi, S.O. Gottlieb, et al. "Incremental Reduction of Serum Total Cholesterol and Low-Density Lipoprotein Cholesterol with the Addition of Plant Stanol Ester-Containing Spread to Statin Therapy." *American Journal of Cardiology* 2000; 86(1):46–52. Lichtenstein, A.H. and R.J. Deckelbaum. "AHA Science Advisory. Stanol/Sterol Ester-Containing Foods and Blood Cholesterol Levels: A Statement for Healthcare Professionals from the Nutrition Committee of the Council on Nutrition, Physical Activity, and Metabolism of the American Heart Association." *Circulation* 2001; 103(8):1177–1779. Plat, J., D.A. Kerckhoffs, R.P. Mensink. "Therapeutic Potential of Plant Sterols and Stanols." *Current Opinions in Lipidology* 2000; 11(6):571–576. De Jong, A., J. Plat, R.P. Mensink. "Metabolic Effects of Plant Sterols and Stanols (Review)." *Journal of Nutritional Biochemistry* 2003; 14(7):362–369. Katan, M.B., S.M. Grundy, P. Jones, et al. "Efficacy and Safety of Plant Stanols and Sterols in the Management of Blood Cholesterol Levels." *Mayo Clinic Proceedings* 2003; 78(8):965–978.

Appendix VI: Expanded Supplement Regimens for Specific Problems Related to CAD

1. Geleijnse, J.M., C. Vermeer, D.E. Grobbee, et al. "Dietary Intake of Menaquinone Is Associated with a Reduced Risk of Coronary Heart Disease: The Rotterdam Study." *Journal of Nutrition* 2004; 134(11):3100–3105.

Index

About the Author

Mark Houston, MD, MS, ABAARM, FACP, FAHA, FASH

DR. MARK C. HOUSTON graduated from Vanderbilt Medical School, completed a medical internship and residency at the University of California at San Francisco, then returned to Vanderbilt Medical Center as chief resident in medicine. Dr. Houston remained on the full-time internal medicine faculty at Vanderbilt University Medical School for twelve years, where he served as medical director of the Executive Physical Program, medical director of the Cooperative Care Center, codirector of the Medical Intensive Care Unit, chief of the clinical section of the Division of General Internal Medicine, and assistant (later associate) professor of medicine.

Dr. Houston is triple board certified, with certifications by the American Board of Internal Medicine, the American Society of Hypertension (ASH) as a specialist in clinical hypertension (FASH), and the American Board of Anti-Aging Medicine (ABAAM). In addition to his medical degrees, he holds a Master of Science degree in clinical human nutrition from the University of Bridgeport, Connecticut.

Dr. Houston is on the consulting editorial board or is a consulting reviewer for more than twenty major US medical journals. He serves as a member of the editorial board and chair of the Medical Advisory Board of the American Nutraceutical Association (ANA), editor-in-chief for the *Journal of the American Nutraceutical Association* (JANA), and member of the Trust and Executive Board for the Consortium of Southeastern Hypertension Control (COSEHC). Dr. Houston has presented more than 10,000 lectures on hypertension nationally and internationally and published more than 150 articles and scientific abstracts in peer-reviewed medical journals, as well as textbook chapters, handbooks, and films. He has also completed more than seventy clinical research studies in hypertension, hyperlipidemia, and cardiovascular disease. Best-selling books he has written include *The Handbook of Antihypertensive Therapy, Vascular Biology for the Clinician,* and *What Your Doctor May Not Tell You About Hypertension: The Revolutionary Nutrition and Lifestyle Program to Help Fight High Blood Pressure, The Hypertension Handbook for Students and Clinicians,* and the *Handbook of Hypertension.*

Dr. Houston was elected as a fellow in the American College of Physicians in 1984 (FACP), fellow of the National Council on High Blood Pressure, fellow of the American Heart Association (FAHA), and fellow of the American Society of Hypertension (FASH) and is a member of numerous medical societies. He specializes in hypertension, lipid disorders, prevention and treatment of cardiovascular diseases, nutrition, clinical age management, and general internal medicine with an active clinical and research practice.

He is presently an associate clinical professor of medicine at Vanderbilt University School of Medicine and director of the Hypertension Institute, Vascular Biology and Life Extension Institute. In addition to being the Hypertension Institute's director, he is also section chief of the Division of Nutrition and director of CME (continuing medical education). Dr. Houston is also a staff physician at Saint Thomas Medical Group and the Vascular Institute of Saint Thomas Hospital in Nashville, Tennessee. He has been selected as one of the top physicians in the United States by *USA Today* and the Consumers Research

Council of American in the fields of hypertension and lipid disorders (dylipidemia).

For more information on Dr. Houston, go to www.Hypertensioninstitute.com. You can reach him at mhoustonhisth@yahoo.com.